SMOKE RISING

Crossing into the Depths of Poverty

Pastor Don,
Continued blessings!
Karen ReMine T.Brockmorton
Matthew 25:40

By Karen ReMine

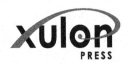
xulon PRESS

SMOKE RISING
Crossing into the Depths of Poverty
by Karen ReMine

Cover photographs by Rob & Dani, *Africa Sunset 1*; Luca Venturi, *Savanna Sunset*.

Interior photographs by Karen ReMine.

Printed in the United States of America.

ISBN 9781498486903

The events portrayed in this book are to the best of Karen ReMine's recollection. While all of stories in this book are true, some names and identities have been changed.

For more information about OMNI, please visit www.omnimissions.com.

www.xulonpress.com

DEDICATION

To my Mom and Dad. Without your loving support and encouragement, the courage to experience these adventures would not have happened.

To my amazing children: Scott, Mark, Daniel, Kimberly, Elena, and Memory. You are my greatest gifts in life.

To my adorable grandson Forrest, you make my world go around.

With love to my dearest best friends Chriss and Gil. You are far better than sisters! 241

To Dr. Henry Maicki, OMNI Medical Director, aka "Jungle Doc." It has been a true honor to serve alongside of you, dear friend.

To those who have compassionately served through Orphan Medical Network International by offering a cup of water to the thirsty, for feeding the hungry, for healing dreaded diseases, praying to rid demons, and tending to the wounds of a leper... you are all angels.

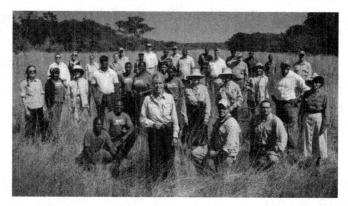

The OMNI team on the Zambian Savana. Photo courtesy OMNI.

Contents

Prologue

I'm in Zambia again. My forty-fifth trip to the continent -- back to the land and the people that so desperately cling to life. I'm in yet another distant village, and I'm feeling exhilarated to do my part to help those in need. It is July, and I am making a home visit to Filishi, the matriarch of a family of several children. Her son and daughter who survived live with her. Her grandchildren did not survive this past year, and their life was cut short like those around her. She could no longer ambulate on her own, or navigate the winding narrow dirt path to our mobile medical clinic beyond the harvested maize field.

Beautiful withered hands and sun dried face showed the lines representing the entire century she had survived. Milky lenses clouded her eyes, allowing only memories of shadows of previous images to enter. She stared long enough into my eyes until her memory showed recognition of our time spent together in the clinic from years past.

When the shadow of my profile cleared in her mind, she smiled and laughed.

She said in her native tongue, "You came back!"

She rolled back on the old stump that was her throne in the dirt as a chicken walked by us -- oblivious of our reunion. Smoke billowed up from the small fire and escaped through the wide slats in the cook hut. Her son watched from a short distance away and held his hand to his mouth as tears filled his eyes. She hadn't smiled in over a year.

I completed her exam after I listened to her heart, took her blood pressure, and took note of her deteriorating condition. Flies swarmed around her legs where body fluids had leaked and fell to the ground.

I presented her with a small gift bag of items: rice for her stomach, a blanket to keep her tiny frame warm in the evenings, analgesics to ease the pain in her old bones, and bath soap as a mere luxury item for this part of the world. I thought my gift would be sufficient for now.

We exchanged our well-wishes as I held her hand in mine.

Her life stretched over one hundred years, surviving malaria, starvation, and the fierce heat of the sun. She outlived her siblings and friends alike, and had witnessed the passing of many. She tells me how one brother was taken by disease. A crocodile attack on the banks of the river claimed her other brother. Only his torn shirt remained.

"When will you take me with you?" Filishi asked.

I looked to her son for interpretation as I could not recognize the Tonga language in the Bemba region of this land.

I paused to give my answer, recognizing her decline and her advanced years. I looked back into the eyes that had witnessed life, death, strength, and endurance in her long life. Her small frame was similar to mine, only withering, fragile, and decaying. I took notice and hesitated.

"When my work is done, dear friend. I'll take you with me when my work is done," I sincerely responded. Heaven would see us both, dear lady.

* * *

Mother Zambia: Good, Beautiful Lady

If Zambia was a human being, she would be a good Christian woman, and a beautiful mother who has grown in wisdom, been widowed and then divorced in her short life. Her high cheek bones and coarse black hair highlighted her dark brown eyes and rich ebony skin. She is humble, kind, and resilient woman who would, and has, sacrificed to protect her children. She has been taken advantage of and abandoned by those who have no respect for her value.

Absolute poverty as well as corruption exist, but this is not Zambia's full story. Life expectancy looms around thirty-eight years, and the infant, neonatal and under-five mortality rates are "unacceptably high," according to UNICEF[1]. As the years go by, however, my lens on Zambia, and the neighboring countries, has become clearer, seeing beyond HIV, malaria, and extreme poverty. Beneath the cover of despair are gentle people, polite and strong. They want what we want, to be healthy, have food, education for their children, and to have dignity despite their living conditions. They seek life and respect. They rely on their own strength and not on government handouts because there are none. They can see joy with little in front of them, and have a faith in God that is stronger than I have seen anywhere. The entire continent

---

[1] "Maternal, Newborn, and Child Health," UNICEF, http://www.unicef.org/zambia/5109_8457.html

steeps in rich culture, are proud of their heritage, and rooted in their faith.

The First Mission

Zambia stamped my passport more than all other countries put together. Thirteen, twenty-eight, thirty-five, forty, and now forty-four long journeys made up multiple entries and Visas on that small, navy booklet. Some passports lay dormant in a bag of VIP papers, retired with a single hole punched through the pages. Russia, Haiti, South Korea, India, Nicaragua were distant runners but mingled within the pages of my precious document that allowed me to cross distant borders and do the work so desperately needed.

The small plane landed on the tarmac; smoke permeated the air so that each of us on this new team could take in the aroma. We had not yet gelled as a unit or knew each other well. I hoped that it would come later as we were there with a purpose and a plan.

Traveling to Zambia requires preparation in advance for your own safety. The CDC recommends getting hepatitis A and B, typhoid, tetanus, and yellow fever vaccinations, because malaria is the leading cause of death in Africa, members of our team take an anti-malaria medication called doxycycline, a low dose antibiotic starting the day of departure and for forty days altogether. I had come prepared and armed at least in the area of disease, but so unprepared really for the permethrin as well, to provide an additional layer of defense against mosquitos. Our team members shower in liquid permethrin, commonly used for lice treatment, which provided a barrier on our skin so that we would not catch scabies from the children we serve. Most importantly, our hearts and souls need the most preparation. Sixteen hours to South Africa, and just a short three hours to Zambia and my husband at the time and three other medical team members are there.

I kept a detailed manifest of the contents of the duffels that were so carefully packed for this mission. The manifest took months to prepare a meticulously logged list of medications, items for the clinics, and all donations for Africa. Drug and regulatory authorities would carefully scrutinize the list before we were allowed passage through customs, so it's detail was essential for our entry. Weight restrictions were strict so we had to be precise with the contents of each precious bag which were stuffed with bandages, syringes, medications, and clothing for the people we hoped to aid. Colored duct tape coded the bags for easy recognition. Red tape meant that there were medications in the bag. Green tape indicated a host of medical supplies, but no medications. White tape was non-medical items such as clothing to give to someone in need or food for the team to survive in any location.

Our bags cleared customs with only a few small items being confiscated. All seemed to be going well for the first couple of hours on the ground until Dr. Chas was arrested. We were informed that he had committed the discriminating crime regarding the preparation of his professional documents. One of his documents was missing his middle initial and he was accused of being a fraud for having more than one name. Three hours later, an intense interrogation, and a payment of a fine, we headed for the northern region of the Copperbelt of Zambia.

The travel time with all going well was seven hours. Our trip took twelve. Checkpoints with armed guards occurred every three hours manned by government police who utilize a shipping container parked at the side of the road, cut in half as an office. I had to assume that full containers were reserved for staff of a higher ranking.

Once in Ndola, we were assigned to the home of Rick and Lauren, a British and South African couple who were living in the city as part of the upper 1 percent of affluent population of the country. Their staff numbered twenty-one nationals, all in uniforms complete with polished shoes and white gloves. We were wined and dined as the "American Team" here to provide medical care to the poor. Fine cognac and South African wines were free flowing along with a five course meal fit for any gourmet connoisseur. The local Embassy staff and professionals who could afford such an evening of indulgence most frequented the restaurant.

Our evening was delightful, and we were anxious to head out to the inner city villages in the morning to set up a mobile clinic. Before we could establish a location, interviews and tours needed to be done to determine the neediest of locations.

Word traveled fast, and soon we had invitations for our team to set up a free clinic. Everyone wanted to be in on the act so to speak.

Campus Crusade for Christ, which was just down the street from the police station and across from the humble offices of Child Welfare, allowed us to use their tiny office for the interviews. The road was a combination of dirt and tar patches, and long forgotten potholes from the rainy season. They served as natural speed bumps for any vehicle or bicycle that happened down this street.

We interviewed all day and saw every combination of Joe and his brother Jim. We referred to them as the "Swindle Brothers." They were here to see what they could get by fabricating what appeared to be the poorest of made up stories, such as, "We have a lot of kids that need food, and we feed them every day."

"Oh really?" I asked, "How many children do you have in your facility?"

"A lot! Just a lot. So, we need your financial support," came the fraudulent reply.

Bogus reports of nonexistent organizations, looking for a quick buck to line their pockets, without giving assistance to help the children of their country. Their attempted hustle was sad and amusingly pathetic at the same time. Most disheartening of all was the fact that there were children within their own village who desperately needed food, shelter, and medical care. Education is essential and would be a dream that very few people there could ever reach.

This training to sniff out corrupt individuals who take advantage of children by proclaiming self-grandeur by creating a facade

13

of care for the poor came in handy years later. I was asked to go to Nicaragua as a consultant to interview a couple who were receiving funds from donors here in the U.S. for their own benefit, while using neighbor's children as local excuses for the money. Large amounts of money came in to their personal account and receipts and records were nowhere to be found. Integrity can't be stolen, but must be earned. Their scam was exposed and justice took its course.

Returning back to our lavish host home after a full day of interviews and chaotic fabrications of need, Rick met us at the door with the latest news. He had a call from one of his "inner circle" of connections that the government paper was going to publish an article in the morning claiming that a U.S. medical team had brought in contraband, and was aligning themselves with the opposing party. The team that they were referring to was us.

It was election year, and a headline like this would sell papers big time, and would get us in even bigger trouble. We had no contraband, and had no alignment with any party. We had no idea who was even running for office, yet alone had any political ties. Our choices were two as Rick put it...Leave the country first thing in the morning and forget doing the work that we intended to do. Bag it, take the loss and leave. Or... go into the deep bush onto tribal land where the government could not have jurisdiction. We were now talking deep bush, deep in the heart of witchcraft country. *National Geographic has not had a spread on this place yet*, I thought.

Not to be a lone ranger, and not to mention that I promised myself that if I went to Africa, I would not go into the bush, I convinced myself that it was much too dangerous. *You could get eaten by something, maybe even someone*, I thought. So I did the right thing and took a vote of the team.

"Who wants to go home and who wants to travel to the unknown?" I asked. I had put it in such a way that it seemed that going home sounded better. We were sitting out under their carport on our duffels, the very supplies that could help those in need. The directions were to close your eyes, and if you wanted to go into the bush, raise your hand. If you wanted to chicken out and go home, don't raise your hand. We all put our heads down and closed our eyes.

"On the count of three raise your hand if you agree to go into the bush," I announced.

"One, two..." I could feel my arm rising as though it was attached to a string in the sky, "... three."

I looked up and all hands were up in the air. No one voted to go home.

It was unanimous; we would leave first thing in the morning for the depths of the unknown. *I may survive this with a lot of prayer.* My other worry, seriously, was that when my mother back in Minnesota finds out, she is going to absolutely kill me!

We are not born with courage, but it is something we should develop. With each step toward courage there is an element of fear involved. Once the fear is overcome courage is strengthened. Without taking the risk to develop courage we lose out in life and fear remains. This was a step in that direction, a step to create courage. Looking back now, I realize that at that moment I had crossed over an imaginary boundary, and everything had changed.

That evening a woman, who appeared very ill, joined our table at our host home for dinner. She wasn't much company or engaging as she laid her head on the table most of the evening and pushed away the food that was presented.

"She has malaria. A tough case of it," our hostess said.

"We've gone to the pharmacy and have some medication for her to take." If she gets started on it right away, the malaria won't be so bad. If she doesn't take it, the malaria could kill her. It has killed so many in these parts." Doreen was to be our new "guide" so to speak, and our means of getting our team out of town and into the deep bush in the morning, provided she survived the night.

The following morning, we left in two older style SUVs, both had seen better days, along with food and bottled water for the journey. Doreen was feeling somewhat better and now only suffered from joint pains and headaches which the medicine, Panadol, seemed to control. It was encouraging that she could stand up now and could drive.

We headed south for about an hour on a two lane tar highway, absent of middle line markers, and speed limit signs. *Not bad*, I thought, and gained confidence that this might be doable. About then we turned to the east and the road became red dirt, full of car size divots created from the rainy season. Oxen carts traveled on this road pulling loads of bundled charcoal for sale in the town. People walked for miles, coming from both directions with what appeared to be no time schedule. It was every man or woman for themselves on this road. Walkers and drivers alike took the path of least resistance as not to not tip or fall into one of the pot holes. Roughly nine women in red and white habits from a religious group I did not recognize walked past us while singing a haunting gospel song in their native language.

Our truck broke down about an hour into this dirt road. Large ant hills rose from the ancient land, abandoned of their habitants and filled with creatures unknown to me. As far as the eye could see, there were dense foliage and no animals or people. Steam arose from under the hood and escaped into the African bush. Our driver, a newly proclaimed missionary from the U.S. had been living in Zambia for a few years, transplanted from her previous home and past. With time and false accreditations, she had somehow convinced one of the tribal Chiefs to donate 1,100 acres of land in the deep bush to her. Her property was our destination that day. I suspect that Doreen was one of those people who had run from something and ran as far as she could into the deep bush of Africa where no one would find her. I found her verbal resume sketchy at best, and her life stories to be even less believable. Her aspirations for her work in Africa were grandiose and lacked planning and preparation.

Doreen claimed that she was a nurse. As a registered nurse myself, I asked a few questions of her that would have been easy to answer and expand upon if that was the case. Her answers were vague sometimes and at other times were clearly erroneous. She lacked the depth of knowledge that a professional nurse would have. Her obvious lack of medical knowledge made it clear that she had no professional medical background.

I later learned that she had worked as a patient aid in a facility years before.

That's great, I thought. We are going into the bush with an imposter who is sick from malaria and no one at home knows where we are. This must be that infamous plan B that everyone talks about. I have come to know that in Africa, plan A never works, and I am not even sure it ever has.

"Does anyone have any gum?" Doreen asked.

"Seriously?" I really thought that this was an odd time for us to be digging into our backpacks for a treat.

"Really, I need a lot of gum so that we can patch up this radiator hose," she explained.

This was my first exposure to African auto repair, and certainly not the last. About two packs of gum later, we were back on the dirt road and ready to now turn south onto what appeared to be a cow path full of randomly positioned rocks. There were massive crooked, tall ant mounds on both sides of the path that were now filled with snakes. Each mound was over eight feet tall and had a large round base. We were warned not to go near them under any circumstances.

My mind raced. Maybe my mother was right. I should have stayed home and not gone to the bush.

That thought prompted the next question, which while I was asking it, took on a higher pitch than my normal voice. "So Doreen, should I be afraid of any animals out here? How about snakes?" I fully expected to hear stories of lions eating the last poor fool who ventured out here, but got instead...

"No, I wouldn't be afraid of any animals at all. You will be safe from those as they aren't many left. They have all been run off or poached years ago. There are some snakes, actually cobras, but I haven't seen one in about a month."

Well, that was a relief, I thought, *maybe I will be all right after all*...interrupting my thought, she said, "You should be afraid of witchcraft though...there is a lot of it out here." Visions of large black iron pots over open fires with me in the soup flew through my mind. Why didn't I think of that? This is worse now than I had previously feared.

"I'll be OK," I told myself. I have to be, as there is no turning around now. I just need to pray harder. And I did.

Just before we turned down a small path marked by a large irregular stone we saw the only creek that ran through the vast rural region of Mpongwe. Women who had walked several miles to this sight were washing their small bundle of clothes in the shallow water that barely moved across the bedrock. Children of various ages were bathing in the same water nearer to the bank.

Dishes were washed in the river using sand from the bottom as an abrasive together with a small piece of plastic that had been torn from the remnants of a corn sack.

As we passed over the narrow bridge on the dirt road, wild pigs from the bush made their way down to the river banks to drink from the contaminated water.

We stopped the truck and walked down to greet the people. Seeing a white person other than Doreen in this area was quite unique for them and I was introduced only as Karen.

"Everyone looks hungry," I said as we shook hands with each person. Children with thin arms and bulging bellies hid behind their mother's shetenge peered from behind the African fabric. "What do we have to give them?" I asked.

We pulled a loaf of bread from the back of the truck and gave each person a single slice of white bread. As we got down to some of the children and the supply of food became less, the bread was split in half and shared until everyone had received something. Smiles were on each person's face and we were rewarded graciously with a curtsy and clapping of the hands out of a sign of appreciation.

I doubted that we would have received the same expression of gratitude handing out a piece of bread back in the States. I took note of the gracious way that they showed their pleasure.

As we were loading back into the truck, the women and children were filling their yellow plastic jugs that once held motor oil with the contaminated water from the creek. The pigs had had their fill and were heading back into the bush as well.

We left to finish our journey deeper into the bush and farther away from civilization.

By the time we arrived at the property, it was dark. Dark in the bush means, black like the inside of a black felt hat in the closet with the lights out. I could see an open fire in the distance, with smoke rising a few feet, then disappearing into the black sky. It reminded me of coming home and having someone leave the porch light on for you. The light from the fire was our beacon to find her hut, a shelter from the unknown possible perils of the bush.

From the glow of the large fire that was burning in the middle of this camp, I could see someone tending to the fire, guarding it actually it seemed. As our eyes struggled to adjust to the extreme darkness, I saw a beautiful white hut with thatched roof about 50 feet from the fire. Behind it - pitch black. I made a mental note to not go back there until morning when I could see what was there.

To the left was a double white hut, again with a thatched roof and a small wooden door that was the entrance into what was Doreen's hut. Just off the fire pit sat a small thatched open structure with four poles made from the trunk of local trees. On each corner chained and ready to attack was an angry dog. Their thinness told us that they were hungry - eager to eat someone or something. These dogs were clearly security for the camp.

"Walk wide when you go by them so they don't bite you," Doreen said. "One of them took after me last month and I had to stop him with a shovel. He learned his lesson but he didn't learn it from anyone else, so I would not go near him."

"Not a problem," I said and took clear note of their viciousness and her warning. Doreen went over to pet each of the dogs and they seemed to settle. I took one step in their direction and they charged at me pulling at the heavy link chain around their necks. *Effective*, was all I could think. Let's hope that the chain is strong...

On the left near the first single hut sat the chapel. The thatched roof circular hut was made from mud and a thin cement-like mixture. Red dirt made up the floor and seemed fairly level until you tried to walk across it. The inside of the hut roof was lined with black plastic to prevent leakage during the rainy season. Bamboo poles created a pattern that ran from the perimeter of the roof to the center where it was tied to a cross beam with heavy twine.

Someone had used some fabric from an African skirt and sewed a simple curtain to hang from a wire stretched across the window secured with a nail on each side. It was a beautiful hut, and the first one that I had ever been in. Little did I know, it became our lodging for that night after the clinic was completed and soon became our home away from home for many years to come.

It was ten in the evening and we had been traveling for days to get here. I thought our day was over, but it was just starting. The chapel doubled as a small area for children to learn how to read and was now the site where 100 locals lined to see our doctors. Our first medical clinic would start as soon as we could unload the duffels filled with medical supplies and set up a makeshift clinic. Our first humanitarian, mash-style clinic was held in the dark of night, with no electricity and fueled by candlelight. Outside the wind whipped through the small outpost throwing dust against the tiny window outlets.

Women with babies lined up first. They secured their babies with a shetenge, or multicolored cloths, wrapped from the back around to the front. Every baby was nursing on the left breast. This, I was told, is so that when the mother needs to, she can swing the baby clockwise to move him onto her back. I often wondered if they ever used the right breast and what problems that it could create if not. This was a technique that I had not taught when working in obstetrics at the Mayo Clinic years before. It would not have worked in our society.

Anyway, a quick adjustment, and a tightening of the fabric in the front and she was ready to move freely with the baby now on her back. Children in Africa travel with their mothers in this fashion until the next baby comes along, usually within a year. They sleep, eat, travel and wet, in the same position for hours. The babies seem content, however, unless someone tries to wake them or move them from this position.

We treated babies, children, women, and men until well after midnight. Trying to establish diagnoses especially on dark skin were a challenge with the limited light. I ran the pharmacy and filled prescriptions of antibiotics, analgesics, and topical ointments by the light of my headlamp and a small candle.

Malaria, pneumonias, TB, HIV, and massive wounds were our challenges of the night. With no medical care within several miles, it was easy to see why the average life expectancy that year was only thirty-two. That means that at sixteen, they were experiencing mid-life!

Simple cuts on the legs running through the sharp elephant grass quickly grew into raging tropical ulcers that would either require amputation, or it would simply take your life. Suffering here is common, and no one is immune. It was a good first clinic and we made our way through all the patients treating their symptoms and curing some simple diseases that would have otherwise killed them. I was convinced that God had put us right where we were needed.

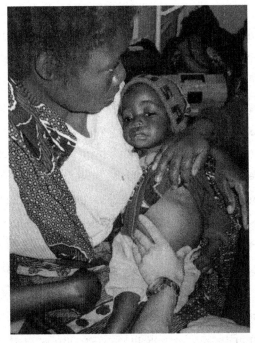

Night clinic at Agape Farm

Sleeping in a hut with five other people on a dirt floor is a challenge to say the least. I managed to turn about every fifteen minutes to keep from molding to the unforgiving contour of the packed earth. Getting up in the night to use the bathroom of which there was none, was tricky. Flashlight in hand, whoever got up would climb across team members, and wander out into the dark of night to find a spot to relieve themselves. I wondered what was in the dark and what crawled on the ground that we could not see on these middle of the night outings. How did the people who lived here survive each night, or did they?

25

Morning comes as soon as the first ray of sun shines through the cloth-covered tiny window. Once outside, I could see where we were and fell in love with the beauty of the Savanna. Just a few yards behind our hut, amber sun, with rising mist from the soil and foliage, filled the air. Birds tweeted, cawed, and cooed in the distance, far enough away so that I could not see them. The Savanna has a peace about it like no other place on earth - magical. Golden bush grass grows about waist high here and bends and flows with the breath of the wind. Trees line the outer perimeter and have a lateral expansion that looks like a water painting where the colors have bleed to each side. I watched as three small birds moved quickly before disappearing. *Smart moves*, I thought, *keeps them from being killed by men with slingshots armed and loaded with stones.*

We knew coming in we would need to bring food and water. Now seeing the area during the day, it is clear as to why - the water is contaminated, and people live on corn grown on their own plots. Water has to be drawn from the creek, where the wild pigs bathe and the women do their dishes. What also came clear is why we had so many complaints of neck pain from the women - they hauled the water they collected in buckets on their heads with their baby strapped to their backs for the long walk home.

An appointed watchman keeps the fire going throughout the night. He pushes the uncut logs from the outside in gradually burning the asterisk shaped wood pile. The team and I waited anxiously for the large pot of water to come to a boil over the open fire so we could have some long-awaited hot tea. Between the five of us, we had to share the one pan of water for our morning mini bath. I had packed bars of soap and small bundles of washcloths for the group. My instructions were absolutely no double dipping. This was all we had for the day. We hung a rope inside the hut to place any clothing we wanted to keep off the ground and to hang our wet wash cloths.

Breakfast was boiled oats that we had carried from home accompanied by a cup of instant coffee or tea. It was hot and filled our stomachs, a necessity to last for another twelve hours until we could return to camp for dinner. No one left food in their tin bowl, and there were no complaints about the breakfast. I loved it.

Later that week, I broke out the good stuff. I had brought corn bread mix and had the assigned cook in the village to mix it up to serve for breakfast. The challenge would be how to bake it with no oven, as there was only an open fire. The woman who cooked for us was quite skilled and created a stone oven placing hot coals at the bottom and covered the sides with pieces of tin from the roof repairs. The biscuits were baked on old tin pans and came out even better than if we would have made them at home. There is a culinary secret involved about eating a meal outside near a fire that makes all food taste amazing!

Before we could finish our meager oatmeal breakfast, people had walked to the location from deep within the bush and were lining up to be seen for their various illnesses and wounds. Our team quickly set up our stations and went to work treating the long lines of tribal families who had not had medical care prior to this day. Mothers with babies on their back stood waiting, often times nursing, but having no food or water themselves during the wait. We treated each patient with dignity and respect and worked tirelessly through the day. The line never seemed to end as people continued to come for care.

Later that afternoon, two men came into the camp struggling to contain and control a young boy who was combative, frothing at the mouth and yelling words that no one could understand. His eyes were dilated, wild and focused on no one in particular, only scanning his surroundings rapidly. He fought to break free, spitting and hissing.

The men laid him down on a large pile of elephant grass that was off to the side of the clinic. They did not let him go. He continued to kick, spit, and scream and could probably be heard into the next village. Our pediatrician and I ran over to him to see what we could do. It appeared that he was having a seizure but we really had no clue what was about to unfold. It was impossible to get any cooperation from the child and the exam was not obtainable.

After taking a short history from the two men that accompanied him, it was determined that he had been poisoned by witchcraft over some dispute between his parents and local witches in the region. Poisoning children for revenge, we learned was common here and often times could be lethal. Our pediatrician was not sure if this could be reversed as he had been in this state of combativeness for almost two days and had not eaten or drank during that time.

We had no antidote for the poison as we did not know what it was that was used. We did feel a presence of evil, and the boy, about ten years, looked as though he was demon possessed. We were out of our league here as far as medical care and were now dealing with the presence of evil and its side effects.

Our pastor on the team and our pediatrician stayed with the boy for a couple of hours and prayed for him and over him. I heard the family and the pastor ask for the presence of evil to leave the boy. It was the closest thing to an exorcism that I have ever seen. The doctor stated that he felt there was nothing more than we could do, and the extent of the poisoning could leave the young boy with permanent brain damage. His seizure activity and his uncontrolled verbal outbursts continued.

Later in the day, the two men escorted the boy back to his farm a few kilometers away to be under the care of his mother. It would not be the last time that we would see him. Joshua was his name.

As the clinic line became somewhat shorter, as in perhaps one hundred more people to be seen, our team was wearing down. We had little sleep the night before, very little food, only small amounts of water, and we had worked all day seeing people who had multiple medical conditions needing care. We had little now, but gave more of ourselves and our supplies. We handed out knit hats, clothing, and shoes to those who needed it most.

Our bus was parked to flank our team and create not only a barrier between us and the rest of the camp, but also a convenient spot to rush into to pull out more supplies from beneath the seats at the rear of the bus from the dusty duffels.

Timing was perfect for the witches to enter. We were tired, day was ending, and their plan was calculating. Chaos had ensued multiple times throughout the day, and we were not educated in this form of attack. As the day neared sundown, the female witches having gone through the line once, came back demanding that their prescription we had filled was not enough, that they had not received a hat, or that they had received nothing at all.

Faces I saw earlier in the day repeated themselves over and over again, and turmoil took over. My endurance and confidence to gain order came through and I made the bold move to ask for the line to stop.

"Chopwa!" (it is finished) I yelled. You could clearly hear the hissing of the women who were witches and their reluctance to stop.

We finally had to throw our supplies into duffels, close up the clinic and pack things into the blue bus which now served as our sanctuary. The clinic was closed. We were now aware of the evil that lurked in this village. I slept uneasy again that night. You could palpate the evil that was there that day. With a bit of planning and organizing, tomorrow we would be ready for the new clinic. I was unclear about how to handle the evil except to pray and be confident that they had no power over us.

Our next clinic was deeper into the bush, passing the vast expansion of the Savanna. We stopped so that we could absorb where we were and take in the absolute beauty that this part of the hidden world held. The path was narrow, and only oxen and cattle carts driven there by young local boys armed with sticks could make use of the treacherous space. Quick sand in various locations had to be portaged by speeding up the vehicle and driving with conviction to pass. This technique didn't always work, and on occasion we all exited the bus to push our way through the sinking sand. Although doing so was exciting, it felt like I was in someone else's reality. The deep bush of Africa surrounded us and had the upper hand!

With the rainy season over, travelers could, for the most part, now pass through the Savanna. There were sections of deep road pockets that our driver maneuvered through with extra care. This time we only had to get out once to push the vehicle, so that wasn't bad. We drove another hour on single paths barely wide enough for our truck. There were a few scattered huts here and there, and people peering out to see the rare passing of a vehicle. Even more rare, it contained white people. We were referred to as a mzungu, or "white face." It's not a very endearing name when you think about it, but it described how we looked to them I guess.

We arrived in a distant village named Chisapa. There were a few buildings made of red brick. None of them had all four sides, and only one had a roof. We chose the three-sided one with no roof, so that we could see who was coming. To the right of the small dilapidated structure, soon to be today's clinic site, stood a huge beautiful tree that we now refer loving to as the "Tree of Life." Its vast trunk stretches four stories into the African sky and has a perfect dome of branches that provide shade for any villager that comes to this area. It is the perceived safety of the tree that provides our shade to protect our team so that we can effectively treat over 600 patients a day.

On this day, however, there were 100 or so people lined up to be seen - some just coming out of curiosity to see what we looked like and what we were doing. Word travels by mouth here as there are no phones or means of communication other than sending a runner with the news. People will walk up to two days to reach the clinic, often times carrying firewood with them to build the night fire along the way. As far as I've seen, no one has carried water or food. They exist on very little.

I set up the pharmacy again expecting today to be a little easier as the medications are more familiar and the majority of people seem to have the same problems. A tall man, maybe in his forties, dressed far better than anyone there, stood near my pharmacy table, looking quite out of place. He offered no indication that he wanted to be seen or that he had any medical needs. He just stood there and watched me work. I didn't mind, however, walking around him each time to get to a patient, or excusing myself to reach for a bottle of antibiotics, became cumbersome, especially when he seemed to have no reason to be there.

I left my post and went over to Doreen who could speak some of the tribal language and asked her to communicate to this gentleman. I either needed him to move, or he would have to start helping me count and load pills into small brown paper envelopes to distribute to patients. A short conversation through a village leader who could speak Bemba and English got my message across I suspected as he started putting vitamins into little envelopes. He caught on fast - observing my actions all morning. All was going well. I had a helper in the pharmacy; we had light, and the day was looking good.

Later that day, I noticed that there were several men holding sticks circling our structure while chanting in their native language.

I asked Doreen, "This is great - interesting. What are they doing out there?"

She replied in a whispered tone, "Those are the male witches and they have been instructed to put a hex on you. The man that you told to get to work, or move out of your way is the head witch doctor!"

I took note of the situation and kept on working as we had many patients yet to be seen.

Our clinic continued until the last patient in line was treated. My new best friend and helper was distant but stayed close to the pharmacy table until we started to pack up the duffels.

Doreen motioned to us that we had to leave before sundown as the route out would be hazardous in the black of night, and would take up to two hours if our navigations went well.

The head witch doctor, along with his entourage, watched every move that we made. There were no goodbyes and no acknowledgement of the medical care that had just been provided.

Our immediate departure was uneventful. Our journey through the deep bush was not.

The winding narrow trails were tough to navigate in the black of night, especially pulling a trailer. We moved slow through quicksand and heavy brush, making our way through the jungle for about thirty minutes when the driver, stopped, and turned around to announce that we had a flat tire.

Everyone turned on their flashlights, exited the vehicle, and shone our lights on the front tire. It was flat, no doubt - so was the rear driver's side, the rear passenger side, and the front of the opposite side.

The night draped its black felt across the jungle. The stars and moon provided a small amount of light on the ground - every little bit helped. A discussion started in the tribal language between the driver and his mechanic.

"We can do this," I said, "Just get out the jack and the spare tires, change them and we will be on our way." Solution.

The two discussed among themselves. Through one of our helpers came the interpretation: "We have no jack, and we have no spare tires."

"Ok, then we go to plan B!" There is always a plan B in Africa as nothing ever works when you try to use plan A. My mind went to the witches. I'm sure they did this.

A school prank, came to mind. *Was this all that they had?*

Our driver and his mechanic created a jack from a large tree limb and rock. Effective and ingenious.

"Everyone off the bus and off load all of the duffels. We need as much weight off the bus as possible to get that tree limb in place," said the driver. Almost ninety minutes later, we were good to go. We climbed back on the bus.

When the engine started, I breathed a sigh of relief, but it was quickly returned when I saw that the bus had no headlights.

"Let me guess, no spare lights either?" I asked.

"We have no spare lights," the mechanic said. He stood to face us. "All hands on deck, so to speak, and bring your flashlights."

We gathered near the front of the bus with three of us on each front window area, shining our lights to create headlights for the bus. The drive through the dense thicket was long. Movement in the bushes told me we weren't alone, but we kept our flashlights in place. We were going to make it out, and no witch could stop us. We arrived back at our destination well after midnight. We had to sleep fast and get ready for the next clinic in the morning several miles away and equally as remote.

The following morning came quicker than our bodies were ready for. We traveled for several hours down a dirt road until we reached our destination - a village farther into the bush and deep beyond the copper mines of Kitwe called Faith Village. Faith was well named. Villagers were proud that with little financial or medical support, they were able to gather assistance in acquiring bandages and basic supplies to tend to the vast needs in this remote village. No other medical care or supplies were available.

Once we finally arrived and were out of the bus, one of the townspeople lead us down a narrow path to a wooden plank placed across the shallow stream. This was the point of Faith's pride. The land had flowing water, and a secure crossing. All of the villagers were extremely poor, and there were no distinctions of class that I could see. There was little food, and poor shelter for most families.

Our team was welcomed and expected to stay in a small, twenty by twelve brick building handcrafted by the locals and mortared by mud from the land. The building contained nothing more than a cement floor and a mesh bin in the corner holding corn cobs barren of their kernels.

Dr. Henry chose a small cement ridge on the back of the wall as his bed for the night probably thinking that heat rises and all would be well. The rest of us settled onto the cement floor with our boots, jackets, and a bed roll. It was cold. I turned every fifteen minutes to keep from freezing and from the harshness of the hard cement. The night was long, and despite the turns there was no comfort to be found longer than a few minutes.

With little sleep and a stiff chilled body, the morning couldn't come fast enough. I got up when the first ray of sun came through the windowless pane and had to walk across the bundled bodies of my team to get out. I headed toward the back of the building to use the grass as my bathroom. On my way back to the confines of our tiny building, I spotted a man by a small fire sound asleep. *Warmth*, was the first thing that came to mind and I felt a bit jealous at first sight.

It was my responsibility to feed the team and get the clinic set up for the day. We were anticipating hundreds who would walk from distant villages to seek medical care. The morning's menu was raisins, oatmeal, and bread, enough for our team. We each had water stowed in our backpacks, but not enough for the full day. We were going to have to replenish our water containers. There were no means to wash up except for our own hand wipes in our bags. The team was accustomed to my travel accommodations and there were no complaints and no whining. I loved that. My team was great.

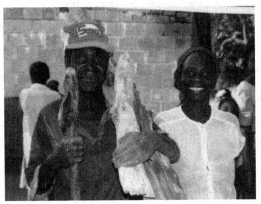

The couple walked two days to get to the clinic.

People had to walk many miles to get to our location. A strong, young couple walked two days with firewood to get to our camp. Their journey was not an easy one, having to find shelter in the bush and gather wood for the journey not only to reach us, but again to travel home. Imagine that in our own country and under those circumstances just to be seen and given vitamins and Tylenol. They will forever remain in my memory.

An Uncanny Meeting

We returned to Agape Farm in Zambia; it was time to form a medical team for the following summer. Our team slept in the same hut again, but this time we were better prepared for the cold nights as we brought small fleece bed rolls and camp pillows. Being so well prepared, I felt like we were stepping up our game a bit.

I rose early to prepare, as I knew this was going to be another busy day. Within no time, the line started to form and soon there were roughly 200 people needing care - many of them coming back again for the second year with obvious trust for our team.

The females in the group who were disruptive and demanding were quickly identified as being female witches sent to distract us from our work and perhaps attempt another hex on our team. We found that we had to remain polite but firm with them, usher them away when necessary, and never ever show fear.

A small young boy came up to me later that afternoon speaking fairly clear English and politely asked for a coat. It was very cold that day, and we happened to have a boy's red jacket in our duffels to be given away. He also asked for a Bible. We had one of those as well, and gave it to him.

"I don't know if you remember me," the boy said to me. "You helped me last year when I was very sick." I looked at him and could not identify him. "I am Joshua," he said. "I heard that your team took very good care of me, but I don't remember it."

The boy although slight in frame seemed healthy and in good shape. He had a smile on his face that for some reason looked familiar.

"Joshua, you are better and I can't believe that you are back!" I said.

His face now free from the demonic glare; his eyes bright and focused. After greeting the doctors in the clinic, he asked to have his picture taken with me. He had a magnetism about him for such a young boy. He smiled then thanked me for the jacket and Bible and left.

We finished our two clinics deep in the Mpongwe region as planned then headed back to town to start the clinics in the destitute compounds. Our first clinic back in Ndola took us to a near dense inner city compound where we set up tables, a few chairs, and unpacked the medications from our duffels.

Mark, my second oldest son, came on this trip as our photographer and while we were treating the sick, would wander through each village capturing the daily living conditions. It was not uncommon of Mark to stop and visit with the locals, ask questions, and take pictures when allowed. He had an uncanny way of making new friends and seemed to adapt easily to the culture.

He made his way to a local shop where coffins were being made by hand, simple, functional, and by our standards - cost next to nothing. The shop never ran out of business as the death rate from HIV/AIDS at that time was high, and treatment was hard to access.

A crowd gathered down the dirt road. The women, dressed in their best clothing, sang and wailed as the men carried one of the handmade caskets on their shoulders toward the cemetery. Another young man had lost his life and was being carried to his final resting place.

Mark noticed, amid all the mourners, a well-dressed woman with a beautiful head-dress and fine leather shoes. Her flawless makeup and nails - painted red - were nothing compared to her smooth, shiny salon groomed hair. She watched Mark for a while, then after the crowd had dispersed from the gravesite, she walked over to him.

"I could not help but notice you, a white man, and here at this funeral. What brings you to Zambia, and who are you working with?" she asked sharply.

"I'm here with OMNI. My mother is the president of the organization; the medical team is here doing clinics for the poor. I am their photographer," Mark answered.

"Well, I would like to meet her. Why don't you and your mother come to my home tomorrow morning for tea so I can learn more about what you are doing?" she continued. "Write down my address and here is my phone number. I will see you tomorrow at ten hours." She didn't wait for a response, she turned and walked away.

"Mark, you have been gone a long time," I said the moment I saw him. "I was getting worried about you. Where did you wander off to?" I asked from behind the pharmacy table.

"I was filming a funeral in town and I met this woman who wants to have tea with us tomorrow at her home," he explained.

"Who did you meet and what does she want to talk about with us?" I asked.

"I met Vera Chiluba, the First Lady of Zambia at a funeral and she wants you to come and have tea with her tomorrow!"

I couldn't believe that we had a tea date in the morning with the wife of the president of the country. President Chiluba was the current residing president, the second to hold office in the country of Zambia since its independence in 1964. This meeting for tea was an honor.

The next morning, Felton our director on the ground, Mark, and another team member and I drove to the home of the president of Zambia. Felton honked the horn at the security gate, and an armed man in a uniform emerged from a small building to the left and asked for our passports and Felton's national identification.

Explanation was offered that we had an appointment for tea with the First Lady. Names were checked on the list, and the gates opened to let our car drive beyond the security gates of their home.

The butler led us toward the living room. My eyes jumped from one place to another - antiques, wood carvings, and gold-plated vases and knick-knacks from other countries filled the space. The home was grand for any country, but was exceptional for Zambia.

"Her lady is finishing her morning preparations and will be with you soon. Please make yourself comfortable."

We sat quietly on the overstuffed sofa and chairs with little communication between us.

I sat and took in the room. Beautiful oil paintings, including a large portrait of the current president, his excellence Frederick Chiluba, adorned the walls. There were items from all over the world that we learned were gifts to the First Lady from other country leaders and presidents.

A well-dressed man sat in the room with us while we waited for our hostess to appear. I was not sure what his connection to the First Lady was, and was not given an introduction. An hour later, the First Lady entered the room. The kitchen maid came behind the swinging door with a silver tray with tea, cups, and small biscuits.

"Tell me about your mission, how you came to be in Zambia, and what motivates you Karen." Commanded Mrs. Chliuba. "I want to know more about your organization and what impact you are having on my people."

"OMNI provides health care, education, and community development to vulnerable children and the poor in a Christian atmosphere of faith," I responded.

"I was asked to come to your country several years ago to assess the medical need that you have here, and since then have developed a mission to provide for those people who have no care or education. Your children are precious and are the future of your country. They deserve an education, and a chance at a better life than the extreme poverty." I explained.

The First Lady was listening carefully and continued to nod in approval as we furthered our conversation. She expressed her approval and her desire for our work to continue.

After the tea and biscuits were finished, we were given a tour of her home, with explanations and stories to verify the various gifts and paintings that hung on the walls.

I found it curious, as we continued the two-hour meeting, that there was no mention of the President in any of the stories or comments. None at all.

President Chiluba was not present. Her only mention of him in the conversation except to say that he was "out" on business. Little more was said of him. *One does not ask about a president unless asked*, I thought.

As we were preparing to leave, Mrs. Chiluba offered a green malachite marble board game as a gift and a hand-painted sea shell with the inscribing, "In service with God" across the outer shell. I accepted the gift with grace.

Before we left the confinements of her yard, the guard opened the front security gate to let a black Mercedes through. A young man stepped out and went to Mrs. Chiluba; he gave her a hug and a kiss on the cheek."

"Meet my son, Castro," said Mrs. Chiluba.

We smiled and nodded. "Nice to meet you," I said. I had read that Castro was one of ten children born to the president.

"He is one to watch and is always in trouble," the First Lady said, casually smiling. "I could take you, Mark, and you could be my son, making you and Castro brothers."

I could see Mark eyeing the Mercedes, the guards, and Castro. *Was he actually considering it?*

"Not a chance," I said with a smile. "He is going home with me."

The young men shook hands and we left. The clinic surely needed us, as it was already in progress. We arrived around noon; there was a lot more work to be done, and I had been away from the clinic far too long.

"Have you seen the headlines of the paper today?" one of the physicians said as soon as we entered the room of our day clinic. "I can't believe that you have not heard about this yet!"

In bold print across the top of the Zambian newspaper was the headline: "President Chiluba wanted for embezzlement."

He was on the run, and the authorities were looking for him. The situation was serious not only for him, but for the country. I doubted that I would be returning to their home anytime soon for tea.

That night, we returned to our lodge to find out that there was no electricity as power shedding was going on to save money in the country. We were relocated to another makeshift lodge, once a home on the other side of town that had a generator.

The accommodations were sparse as well as the food and its quality. Each room shared a bath that had bouts of electrical currents running along the pipes. If you touched the hot faucet we would get a shock. If you touched the cold faucet you would get a bigger shock.

The clothes that were washed were hung on metal lines outside my room that I shared with Gil and one of the female doctors on the team. There were chickens and one very annoying rooster that woke up each morning at 4:30 making his loud crows under each window of our lodge until he had successfully woken everyone up well before we needed to be. Rumors among our team started to spread that his life was going to be cut short and rightfully so.

On the last day that we stayed there, dinner was unknown chicken parts and boiled potatoes. I didn't eat much that night.

The Seventh Son

"The world today is hungry not only for bread, but hungry for love; hungry to be wanted, and to be loved." - **Mother Teresa**

There is no room in this world for apathy. Apathy makes hearts stagnant and lethargic for the needs of others. Each of us can do something somewhere for someone. I have always thought of the world as mine and yours. We are citizens of the world not just a resident of the country that we live in. With social media and live television, we can see the needs of the globe and hopefully will feel the responsibility to be moved to act with compassion.

We learned through our work that the needs of the orphaned and vulnerable must transcend our apathy that preserves our own comfort zone. Each of us is capable if willing to respond.

I'm beyond passionate when it comes to doing something about the suffering caused by starvation, the wasting caused by disease, and the lack of hope secondary to a lack of education and the combination of any of the above. I am moved to do something to help. Any one of these on its own robs a child of a future. Cumulatively these cruelties can deprive a child of their life. Everyone deserves the basic necessities that sustain a human's existence. Everyone can do something. I am determined to do the same and to wake up hearts where apathy has caused sedation.

To understand it, one has to understand poverty. Not the poverty that we think of here, such as a broken down car, or a lack of a color television, perhaps over-worn clothes, and a limited amount of food for dinner. To understand it, we have to realize that the poverty that robs one of their lives is absolute. Extreme poverty means that the family lacks those very basic things that sustain life, such as clean water, shelter, healthcare, and food - any food. There is no income, as there are no jobs to be had anywhere within walking distance or beyond. There are no government programs to fill in the gaps that poverty creates. It is understanding that zero plus zero is still the same sum of the two.

The family structure is interrupted by the death of a parent, or often times both. The children are left to survive on their own with no resources. Grandparents in the winter of their lives raise grandchildren with no income. Often times the income earning generation is dead. Children care for children or are head of households. School becomes only a pipe dream or a hit or miss event.

Children without parents who live in an area of extreme poverty are vulnerable to the downward spiral of life threatening side effects. They suffer from malnutrition, lack of health care, no education, and are stripped of a life beyond a couple of decades if they are lucky. They have no voice to protect them. In the cities, small children become victims to predators and often times the deathly grip of drugs that numbs the pain of their hunger. We can do something about it, and we can, and do make a difference in their lives.

Even in an area where there are free government schools - uniforms are required. Twelve dollars is more than the average income for a month. Food or a uniform? What would you choose? Which child do you choose gets to eat today? Who goes without until tomorrow or the next day? The agony of these decisions is painful to watch, and even more painful to make.

Memory was the seventh son, and the last to be born to a couple who lived in the shadows of the copper mines in Kitwe. Seven sons were born to them in the most adverse conditions. Food, shelter, healthcare, and safety were not available. Birth control is also not within reach and not within concept. Life is life as it is. Babies are born. Babies die. Life is a struggle to exist. There are no means of getting away; no education to lift you out of poverty. There is no hope. Life and death happens every day. Survival modes are inherent.

Smoke billows from the mines and creates a dense fog of pollution. Lung diseases are common in that area, topped by malaria and HIV. Poverty is everywhere and is etched on every face.

Not far from the mine, in the heart of what is called the Chambishi Township, lies a boundless slum that is home to many of the mine's workers and their families. From the base of this impoverished village a hazy silhouette of the Congo hills can be seen in the distance. Memory and his brother lived in a small mud shack located on the right side of a rain washed dirt and rock road. Few have electricity, and there is no running water.

Nine people lived in a twelve by sixteen-foot structure. The nuptial bed is shared with several children, while the older ones sleep on the floor just outside of the flour sack hanging by threads that doubles as a door. Toilets are holes dug in the ground surrounded by bamboo and elephant grass bound by twine somewhere on the street. Chickens and a few small goats roam among the shirtless, shoeless children that populate this slum. In the rainy season, water flows like a mighty river down the rocky dirt road dividing the rows of shacks from each other. Walking the road is unsafe. Trying to drive a vehicle through the uneven rock laden road is almost impossible.

Makeshift three-sided shacks selling local beer to blaring Zambian hip hop soundtracks tend to attract young men like flies. Local unpasteurized brew helps to ease the pain of poverty. Alcoholism and all that accompanies this debilitating disease affects most families in one way or another. More babies are born with no means of caring for them except for young girls who are destined to be their mothers.

The entrepreneurial alcohol business sits alongside a pit filled with rubbish, a common sight in the township. Ditches filled with garbage and stagnant rain water cook in the afternoon hot sun. Since the government rarely collects the trash here, the residents have taken to digging these pits and tossing in additional deposits themselves. There is an increase of flies and mosquitoes, as well as their attendant diseases. More than 25% of annual mortality in the Copperbelt region is due to malaria; one in five people there have HIV. In the township itself parasites multiply alongside the desperate prostitutes who know no other business. The numbers of fatal diseases here are even worse. More babies are born, and struggle to live, and eventually die at a young age.

Next to the large dark gray mine is a small private clinic owned by the mine. The hand constructed "Morgue Entrance" sign can be clearly seen from the road, and is the most frequented site on the facility. The wooden frame had clearly been inscribed in someone's own hand using a crude brush and paint. The letters were uneven but clearly conveyed the information for entrance provided that you could read English. Families bring in loved ones with little hope of bringing them out alive. Mourners, wailing and singing hymns, leave the facility accompanying the clothe-bound lifeless bodies on their final journey to be buried in a local cemetery. Single wooden handmade crosses etched by hand mark the simple graves. Scattered hand cut flowers from the fields adorn the dirt mound.

In addition to being born into another generation of poverty, Memory was physically branded with a severe club foot on the right side. In certain societies this deformity that comes across as a weakness to others who may want to take advantage and often do. His foot curled under so severely that he had to walk on the top of his foot which now doubled as his sole. Shoes were impossible to wear, and his gate was cumbersome and painful. Because he used his left foot to run or hop on when jumping from any elevation, the right lower leg showed signs of significant atrophy from lack of use. He was visually noted for being different and deemed as a target for someone to abuse.

Memory was orphaned at the age of two along with his six older brothers. His mother Jane, died when he was only 3 months old, and his father, Green, died when Memory was a toddler of only two. He has no recollection of either parent and remembers nothing of their presence or what they looked or sounded like.

Both parents died of malaria, a treatable disease that in Africa can evolve into a death sentence when you do not have the $3 needed for the treatment. Malaria is the number one killer in the continent of Africa leaving a sea of orphans in its wake. Memory is a name given to the youngest child when there has been a death in the family, and can be given to either gender. With each name, there is a story of loss. Loss is common here to every family, and rarely does anyone discuss it or bring attention to it.

Death is a part of life. It just seems to come more frequently here and far too early in their existence. It amazes me how fragile life is here. Loss of life is a daily occurrence and seems to happen more frequently the more you travel deeper into the villages. Large families dwindle to a few. Mothers, sisters, sons, and fathers die far earlier than what we are used to especially when you take into account that life expectancy when we arrived in Africa was thirty-two. Despite a high majority of infant mortalities and post-partum deaths, Africa considers itself to have no orphans. Everyone is connected to someone in their family no matter how distant the relative.

In the Zambian culture, there is no word to describe a cousin, or an aunt, or uncle. If your father's brother is older than your father, he is considered to be your "big father", and the same scenario if he is younger, now becoming your "small father." If your brothers' or sisters' children live with you, they are your children and are treated equally in that respect. Memory would be cared for by his brothers, all older, not orphans, but had no mother or father in his culture. The family profile was common, but not ideal.

The streets, where Memory ran free with no supervision were lined with good intentions or so it seemed. Small shopkeepers sold their wares. A few buckets of fritters made from corn, eggs from the local chickens, and whatever small items one needed to exist could be found. Many of the food items were sold on small mats on the ground that were maintained by women with babies on their backs, trying to make enough money to survive day by day.

When no one was looking, Memory, and sometimes his brother Dow, would steal a piece of bread, and run with his irregular gate, hopping on his good foot and keeping the club foot elevated. Because of his deformity children would throw stones and call him names. Growing up with no one to answer to and no one to care about his safety or his emotional well-being wasn't easy. He was his own boss and he knew it no other way.

Memory's body craved nutrition; the best he could figure out was to eat dirt from the roadside. It filled his stomach and in a way unknown to him, provided some form of sustenance in the form of minerals, no matter how slight - it was better than nothing. Soil contains iron, zinc, and calcium in small amounts. It fills the stomach and eases the hunger pains. In some cases, consuming dirt rids the stomach of parasites often found in the contaminated water. Memory has had a few diseases except for malaria - the number one killer of the continent.

The same dirt, when mixed with water, creates a clay-like substance used to make amazing toys that resemble coveted items of the world. A rectangular shape, dried with the addition of a small piece of wire, turns into a mini boom box, that can transform any day into one filled with music in your mind. Tattered shreds of plastic, when bound with string, become a soccer ball creating endless hours of kicking and running with friends. Discarded milk cartons transform into buses and cars, and with a bit of wire and discarded lids, wheels make the object even more enjoyable. The possibilities are endless with just a few pieces of garbage and creative imagination.

Being double orphaned leaves you extremely vulnerable to the grips of poverty. Imagine seven boys, with no income and no means of getting food. With no money, there was no possibility to attend school, which made it difficult to get a job. Survival, daily and long-term, became a challenge every day. Memory became his own boss and navigator of the world as his brothers had their own challenges and need for individual survival.

Memory has a recollection of his oldest brother signing him up for school, an educational opportunity offered to children of the mine's employees. The small school took place in a tin building at the base of the mine. Memory's oldest brother sent his noon meal which was a piece of bread wrapped in brown paper. Sometime during those first few hours, someone stole the bread and when it came time for Memory's first meal of the day, there was none to be had. He left the school that day, walked home and never returned.

At the age of four his older brothers realized that they could not feed him or care for him any longer and made the difficult decision to walk many miles to their auntie's house who also had children of her own. Determined to help him survive, they left him to the care of a relative who they barely knew.

Without anyone to check on his welfare, the cold-hearted aunt made a conscious decision to withhold food from Memory, and feed her children in his presence instead. He was made to watch them eat their food while sitting on the floor across the room. He would go to bed hungry, and feared for his life, as her disdain for the burden of another child grew. To make matters worse, when she felt he was asleep on the floor, she would walk by and kick his head, perhaps hoping to create an injury that he would not survive, but Memory grew aware of her evil aggressions and was always on guard.

Running away seemed to be the only option, which he tried several times to accomplish, however was found and dragged back to the house. On a hot afternoon one summer, the heartless, evil aunt dragged Memory down to the creek and held his head underwater. One of the older children witnessed the murder attempt and pulled the woman away.

The need to be with his brothers overcame the distance for him to find his family again.

Chris and Luxem, the oldest brothers visited Memory a short time after his placement at the house of their mother's sister. It was clear that Memory was suffering more than he would be with them, and made the decision to take him during the night from his abuser. They would find some way to care for him. They had to, he was their brother.

Luxem, unemployed and hungry, was wandering the streets of Kitwe, when he met a woman from the U.S. Her story was that she was in Africa trying to establish an orphanage for boys in the deep bush, tribal regions. He was offered placement at the rural region facility called Agape, the Greek word for *unconditional love.*

The 1,100-acre camp, gifted to her from the tribal chief in that area on the condition that she would help the orphans on his land, was untamed, hard to obtain, and deep in the bush of Zambia. The rich soil had not yet been developed except for a few foot paths that meandered through the ant hills and some growth of elephant grass. Trees grew tall and touched the deep blue palate of the African sky. Few people had ever been there except for the native population- and now us.

With funds from the chief and from donors in the U.S., Doreen built her small camp deep within the jungle and far from civilization. Her home now consisted of two round huts joined by a small passageway connecting a space for a bedroom and a space for a table on the other side. Broad timbers from the forest created the cross beams over her bed. Her inky black cat would slink across the wooden beam with panther-like movements. The cat, larger than most domestic cats, resembled the big cat panther in many ways. I often thought that there was more resemblance to the larger animal making this particular one a cross of wild and domestic. The feline beast was kept to kill the rats that scurried across the floor looking for food.

A well was dug to reach the deep clean water that flowed under the earth. Doreen's staff, made up of local villagers, would lower large buckets attached to ropes deep into the ground and retrieve the life giving waters from below. The water collected was then boiled for drinking and cooling water.

A small garden held infant plants; maize grew in tall rows in the back and remnants of corn cobs stripped of their yellow buds scattered the ground behind the house. Just up a narrow path sat a small outhouse with a wooden door. With no electricity, candles became the main source of light. They were, however, hard to come by and were only sold in town which was a two-hour drive on rough dirt roads - so candles were burned only when necessary. The only illumination at night came from the stars that layered the heavens here like diamonds.

This camp would eventually become the home for eighteen vulnerable little boys who had no residence of their own. These were children who had lost family members, had no stable home, no source of food, or an education. They were statistics doomed for a sad outcome in life.

Two hot meals a day and a roof, with no leakage, now covered his head. Life was more tolerable and less unpredictable. It was something he had not had if ever in his life. He kept Memory in his mind even though they were separated in distance and void of communication.

It was a cold afternoon in the middle of the African winter when Doreen drove into the camp while our team tended to patients. Luxem and a small boy wearing an oversized jacket and knit hat emerged from the back of the truck. The boy wore no shoes, which easily revealed his deformed right foot. He lacked a smile or any facial expressions that a child would wear. The void on his face matched his dark sad eyes.

Our team held back the exclamation that we felt in our hearts to see this withered tiny foot that curved inward and under. The top of his foot had several new and old callouses. The inner sole could not see the light of the sun as it was curled into itself. His right calf appeared crumbled due to lack of use. The pediatrician examined his foot, and knew even before he started the exam, that there was nothing we would be able to do for this child here in Zambia. A foot so severely deformed would require extensive surgical reconstruction and rehabilitation to achieve any functional limb. There were no clinics in Zambia that could offer such surgical expertise and without it, life with a severe neglected clubfoot, would be a lifelong challenge.

There are times in my life when events move forward that is so enormous, and I know that I am only the conduit to make it happen. God has incredible plans for us - plans we could never create or master on our own. Memory was just one of them.

Preparation to get Memory to the U.S. was extensive and laborious. Memory came to Agape Farm so that we could enhance his medical well-being with good nutrition and security for his safety. I returned to Agape with a small medical and building team as we awaited an overseas container that we had shipped from the U.S. four months earlier. Rick, our building director, had organized a small team to build the two homes for the boys on the farm's land. The container had been loaded with medical supplies as well as building supplies including lumber, tresses, mattresses, and furniture for the homes for the boys.

As international work has it, the container was lost about three weeks into the journey from Michigan to New York and was then dry docked in Israel where a strike. Over a month passed with multiple e-mails and phone calls to our shipping agent to ensure that the container would once again head to its destination of Zambia.

All seemed to be going well until the container made its way through Zimbabwe from the Durban port on the back of a truck where it got held for ransom. The trucker requested $4,000. The amount was more than he would have made in a year with his work. We held out, like a card game, hoping that we could sustain and endure the bribe. No money was exchanged and the shipment was released to our destination. Our team was in Agape and the container was somewhere crossing the African continent.

As God would have it, the extreme remote dirt of the hidden bush of Zambia began to roll and from the dust, a semi-truck pulling a container that originated in Michigan emerged.

Villagers gathered and our team and those that we did not know cheered as the truck came closer. It was a miracle. The items that were gathered over a year ago, packed and prayed over, then lost in Israel and released through the vast continent of Africa arrived! This was small in comparison to the journey, but the lock that was placed on the two hundred twenty thousand-pound container had no key, and the container had to be offloaded to the ground with only man power. The sun was starting to lower into the horizon and the driver of the truck was anxious to do an offload. Rick gathered several of the strongest men from the village to put together a plan to lower the rectangular steel box to the ground.

The plan of action was formulated soon long ropes were attached to the end of the container and secured around a large tree that stood a few feet away from the project site. Logs that had been timbered and cut for firewood were hand carried by the locals to the end of the truck bed. Grinding metal echoed in the air as the driver pulled forward causing the rear of the container to tilt slightly making its way to the makeshift log roller beneath. The only light that assisted the process was the small fire that the truck driver had built earlier to cook his corn for his evening meal.

Each surge forward strained the truck's engine and progress came in staggered increments until the final drop of front end of the container slammed onto the red clay below. Rolls of dust billowed out from under and around the steel box as the tribal villagers cheered and the women cried out with signs of approval. With a few brief words of gratitude and handshakes here and there, the truck disappeared into the darkness.

Zambian people are resourceful and for that I love their spirit. Rick handles his men like he handles the workload – fast, efficient and with strength. He is an incredible leader that can manage and make the tough situations look like child's play. One of the men, using a crow bar of sorts, pried open the lock.

In all of this excitement, and now dark with no lights, children gathered around the amazing structure of steel that contained unknowns to them. Excitement bounced on the air waves. A group of boys came from out of the tree line and gathered around me. One child stood out from all of them. I recognized Memory from our previous clinic and despite our brief meeting and encounter, he stayed close to me, letting other children know of his familiarity with this white woman. It was noticeable and his presence tugged at my heart. Who was this child and why was he and I brought together in this serendipitous meeting?

Children living without parents and fending for themselves is a sad and common reality in Africa. Having to steal, beg, or scavenge for food is a survival skill that unfortunately is ramped. There are few, however, that have the skills or knowledge to earn money legitimately.

One day when Felton and I were in town with the intention of buying medications for the children in Agape, we saw just how real that statement truly is. We parked on a city street where many of the street people linger, hoping that a hand out of money from parked cars will sustain them. Young children approach such cars, with hands extended, faces contorted, and bellies empty. That particular day, a young boy about ten years approached me with a small wooden step stool handmade with four legs secured by a cross bar of wood. The wood was sanded, and stained, and the seat had been broken, and glued so that it did not appear to be damaged.

"How much is the stool?" I asked Felton.

"Don't bother with him. He is just a beggar," he replied.

Before we could walk away, the little boy indicated to Felton that the stool was four U.S. dollars.

"I want to buy that stool," I said.

"It is too much money. I will make him go away," Felton said.

"No, tell him that I will buy that stool and I want him to not have to beg any longer today," I instructed.

I knew the moment the boy understood, as a huge smile made its way across his little face.

I paid for the stool then took a few moments to admire it - a far greater treasure than anything $4.00 has ever bought me. It still sits in my office today, and I sit on it from time to time to remember that little boy.

Billboard signs now line the streets of most cities urging people like me to not give money to the street children as they will most likely be controlled by adults who take the money from them. The stool, however, represents a tangible treasure for me to ensure that I will remember that child forever. I prayed that the money filled his stomach and eased the pain even for just a day. He could have been Memory on that street, but he had a different future ahead of him.

Less than a year later, Memory flew home with the OMNI team to Michigan along with an interpreter. Both stayed at our home in preparation for complicated surgery that lasted seven hours. Memory's surgery took place in a large hospital in Michigan under the stellar care of an orthopedic surgeon who amazingly reconstructed his foot - moving, rearranging bones, and creating a functioning appendage.

Memory approached me one morning in the kitchen - his favorite room in the house - and asked, "What should I call you?"

"What would you like to call me?"

"I would like to call you Mom," he replied.

Six months later, the interpreter flew home and Memory stayed behind, determined to become a permanent part of our family, and the sixth child for my husband and me.

His life changed from that moment on. Opportunities to thrive were given, education was a daily exposure, food came in abundance, and clean clothing was always available. The most important to him and to us, was the presence of a family that loved him.

"What happens if you don't eat?" I asked him one day after several months with us. I fully expected to hear the description of hunger and how your stomach hurts, you feel light headed and weak, but his answer was very simple and short.

"You die," he replied. His statement was shockingly profound.

Adoption was the obvious solution to permanently providing Memory with a family who loved him and could ensure a viable future. The process was lengthy and creative as there are very few adoptions done nationally or internationally in Zambia.

Mounds of paperwork, home studies here and in Zambia, and court hearing after court hearing, the adoption process inched forward. Because Memory was a minor and was in the custody of his oldest brother, a legal document had to be drawn up that granted his relinquishment to us. Chris, the oldest of the seven boys who was Memory's legal guardian, had to be located and brought to my attorney's

63

office in Ndola to sign the official papers. The task of finding him was a difficult one, as there are little resources to locate someone who has no address or phone - all had to be done word of mouth.

I traveled alone on this trip with two other board members. Cutter had to find out where he worked, ask people on the street if they knew of him or his brothers, and hope that someone would know of him. The process took us two days, and we were fortunate to find a man on the street who knew that Chris often parked his cab in front of a grocery store hoping to catch fares as they left the store.

We located him and through an interpreter, explained what needed to be done, and how Memory would soon begin the process of having a stable family through adoption. Explanations had to be repeated and after a long discussion, Chris agreed to ride with us to Ndola, a town he had never gone to and present himself in front of the attorney who was handling Memory's case.

Chris entered the office and stood straight against the wall across from the attorney's desk. When he was asked to give his name, he slid down the wall and knelt on the floor with his eyes fixed downward displaying respect. His demeanor was a lesson in extreme humility with respect to the attorney who was his senior and far more educated than he. Tears ran down his face as he signed the document of relinquishment fearing that he would never see his brother again. Through the interpreter there seemed to be no words that would give him the comfort and assurance that he needed to sign his brother's care to us.

"I'll take good care of him, and he will be my son," I assured him. "You will hear from me each time I come into the country, and I will bring pictures and word of his well-being."

Chris signed an "X" on the line where his first and last name should be since he could not read or write. He understood the implications of his signature and for the first time looked into my eyes for confirmation that he had done the right thing for Memory. I saw him through the tears and neither of us had words that were adequate. We both remained silent, but connected now through the life of this small little boy.

The court appearances were fascinating and different each time. I was required to go before the judge and along with my husband declare our intentions. Since I traveled there alone, I had team members stand in with me in court and acknowledge the intent of my wishes to adopt this child.

The judge in Zambia granted Memory's adoption, a rare and unusual event in a country that has no formal adoption process. Adoption papers were filled out along with a birth certificate that was created by the courts. They gave him his new formal name, a new birthdate, which was the same month, but different day and to our surprise a different year than when he was born. U.S. citizenship was eventually granted here as well, after a couple of years passed according to the current laws.

I now have ten sons, counting my seven in Africa. When I am in Zambia, I am referred to as "Bana Memory," or the mother of Memory, a title of which I am proudest.

I can't help but wonder, *What God-given gifts of grace are given to children or adults that give them the strength, will, and skills to survive the most adverse conditions?*

Together in Mission

Our family moved from one state to another more often than I'd like; our sixth move was approaching due to the changing of my husband's job. I was not sure how OMNI, our marriage or I would survive the move. I had left my friends, church, and home five times before, and I would have to do this again soon. The tension of moving played heavily on us.

The first evening of our arrival my husband announced that we needed to attend a dinner where I met an amazing woman who ended up being one of my dearest friends. I had learned to be prepared for short notices and had a dress packed next to the parakeet cage and the bed for the Beagle. Everything had fit nicely into the back of my car and survived the long drive from Ohio. The dinner was in a large complex downtown and I happened to meet Gil within a few feet of the entrance as we entered into a sea of unfamiliar faces, names unknown, and layers of corporate hierarchy.

She asked where I worked, hoping to strike up a conversation of some common ground. I could see by the expression on her face that she did not expect to hear me say "Africa." She was a registered nurse as well and the bond quickly formed.

"I want to go to Zambia with you and work," she said. I gave her my business card, fully expecting like many others, there would be no forward motion in that regard after our meeting.

Gil did sign up though. Being an RN, she came not only with work experience but also compassion, which she brought with her on every mission trip. It's been nine years now of endless dedication, and fundraising. Together we organize then pack for the entire medical mission every year.

"I get it now," she said one day after we returned. "You have been doing this pretty much on your own, and it's authentic. I'll be here as long as you will have me on the team." And God brought another best friend into my life through missions. Christine, or "Chriss" as she prefers to be called, became an equally precious friend that same year having met her at a mission's fair at our church. Together their friendship and constant support of the mission has been priceless. Their constant support and presence holds a candle next to none. I am so blessed to have them in my life.

In our church, yet another person comes into OMNI's life with dedication to missions. He took us all by surprise as our church was seeking an associate pastor.

As the search process goes, candidates from all over the U.S. may apply for a position within the Synod and through a lengthy call process, he or she is invited to apply for the interview. Such was the case several years ago. I had no idea that the person chosen for the position would become an integral part of our mission life. He was born and raised in Zambia and had come to the U.S. for seminary training and to minister to the people of America, at the same time my team was developing a ministry to serve the people in Africa.

A meeting was arranged for me to meet him and discuss the work that we did in Zambia, his country of origin. Out of respect for him and his culture, I knew that this meeting would require certain protocol on my part.

I would need to wear a skirt that fell somewhere below my knees, yet not to the floor. I would greet him with a proper curtsey, eyes cast downward. At the same time, I would include the Zambian handshake that of which is extending your right hand to shake while your left hand grasps the right arm just below the elbow. This gesture was a sign of respect of which a man of this position deserved. If one were to be of a lower status of education in Zambia, kneeling or squatting down next to the person as they sit to ask a question upon entering the room shows acknowledgement of importance and esteem.

He grew up in the tribal region that our team worked in and was here in the U.S. as a product of the efforts and compassion from missionaries serving his people. Compassion is defined as the feeling of empathy for others. It is the emotion that we feel in response to the suffering of others that motivates a desire to help. He was an example of the ripple effect that can change lives forever. That momentum of compassion can perpetuate itself for generations. What a powerful way to change the world. It penetrates even the hardest of hearts and strengthens the weakest bodies.

Working in missions all over the world creates many interesting combinations of people. I have always believed that missions are good for everyone, however, not everyone is good for missions. Some people can down right destroy the best team that has been put together simply by being and indulging in themselves. Then you add sleep deprivation, change in routine, strange food, and a team monster is born, hell bent on being the monkey wrench in everything you try to do.

There seems to be a draw for those that need some type of adjustment in their lives and feel that going on the other side of the world will give them something that is perhaps missing in their life, like sanity. We have had a few "red flags" as I refer to them somehow slip through the interview process and end up becoming our work around overseas. It's always interesting when a team is willing to put all of their spending money together to buy a one-way ticket back to the U.S. for that incredible misfit on the team. It has never happened, however, but I have spent many times having serious conversations about attitudes and how to adjust them to make them work. Not all of these attempts are successful, so we place the bandage on difficult behavior and get by.

On the other hand, there are those people who when you first meet them, you know immediately that this person has been sent to you and to this mission as a blessing.

I had been working in Zambia, Africa for eight years, and had experienced meeting tribal chiefs, working with the extreme poor, traveling in unknown regions, and facing what I thought would be demise. All the time, I was engrained in the indigenous population and wanted to go back. I was put on this earth to serve the poor truly loving this work and the people.

A rural tribal region that is home to the Bemba tribe Mpongwe and its surroundings found me to be a frequent visitor. Getting there on the ungraded pothole-filled dirt roads was not easy and always had multiple mishaps and adventures in our journey.

By chance a few years back, I had been asked to meet with the second largest landowner Chieftainess in the country of seventy-two tribes. She rules several thousand acres and had been voted into her royal position after her brother died. Lineage was essential for the inheritance of the crown. She wore it well, including carrying a scepter made of ivory and the tail of an elephant. The elephant hair portion of this royal item including the ivory was constructed by hand and was not allowed to be carried by anyone but the chief. It was out of bounds to anyone and forbidden to touch. The hair from the elephant, even though centuries old, had broken off and was probably about two feet shorter than its original state. She held the ivory handle in her right hand, stroking the elephant hair with her left. Mark, my second born son was with us on one of the meetings with her and asked if he could touch it. Her answer was swift and blunt. "No! You will melt!" I thought of Dorothy and Toto defending them against the wicked witch. Melting was another fear that I had not thought of. I could add that to the snakes and large animals that loomed in my mind as dangerous.

Her smooth ebony skin, which was regularly bathed and oiled, was only one of her beauty traits. Her stature straight and confident, spoke volumes of her upbringing. Her dark brown hair, tied neatly upon her head so that her crown could be placed with security, surrounded a flawless round face, full from living a privileged life. On her right wrist hung a thick round bracelet made of pure ivory, possibly from elephants that at one time roamed the beautiful Savanna. On her left hand a heavy band of gold, not known to many in this country, signified her marriage to her husband.

I couldn't help but admire her long deep blue dress that was partially concealed by her red royal robe, trimmed with bands of black fabric on the front and the sleeves. A crown made from red fabric adorned with braiding and an insignia of her tribe sat perfectly and firmly atop of her head. When she spoke, her voice was strong and her English clear. When angered, her voice dropped in tone and grew more stern with every syllable. Chieftainess Melanbecka was a woman who demanded respect - which I did not doubt was received at every encounter on every occasion.

As a chief, she can demand whatever she wants and it will usually happen. Cross her and you will be verbally chastised and driven from the vast land that she owns. She is a woman of faith and believes in God and His grace that is now upon her and her land.

It is customary and politically correct to bring a gift from each person to present to the chief. Over the years, our gifts have varied from a crate of oranges, which is considered a delicacy to live chickens that we purchased on the roadside from a vendor who harbored the poor foul in a handmade wire basket doomed not to see the next light of day. The chickens rode on our bus in the front passenger side and were, for a short time, in their lives considered "free range chickens." I am not fond of riding with a live chicken and would not recommend it to other foreign travelers. Anything with wings will take flight and flying chickens in a bus is a road hazard in my opinion.

The following year, we visited the chief in her "palace" - her home that is protected by several guards and servants. The red dirt road leads to a small hut near the gate where we parked our vehicle. "You are to wait here until the Chieftainess is ready to receive you," came the instructions from the guard.

Two hours later, we were allowed entrance into the palace grounds and were instructed to enter with the respectful heads bowed, and hands clapping together in sessions of three, three times. This clapping would announce our arrival and shows respect to her heinous.

The Chieftainess has the first right to speak and we are not to speak unless spoken to. I felt like I was in school a century ago but of course complied with the rules.

Once we were received, we were allowed to look up at her and answer any questions that she might have. It was an awkward meeting coming from such diverse cultures but it worked. She had warmed up enough to our team to ask for her next gift!

"I want a tiara," she proclaimed.

My mind raced. *Where in the world would I find a headpiece that would be sufficient?* I looked up at the pillbox-shaped hat on top of her head, made to match the royal red robe.

Would she like to remove the hat for the tiara, or how would that work? I wondered.

Once back in the U.S. and preparing for my return trip to Africa. I scoured the accessory cases at local bridal shops and finally purchased a tiara fit for a queen. It was perfect, and even included a nice gift box. I was so excited to bring this symbol of royalty to her that I could hardly wait for the next mission trip. It needed something more. I pictured kings and queens that wore long velvet robes of rich colors - burgundy and deep purple.

The eighth grade formal winter ball popped into my mind like an old movie. I wore the most beautiful velvet floor length deep burgundy skirt. My mother made it for me to save money and to get the exact skirt I wanted. For whatever reason, I had saved it for thirty years in a box just waiting for this very moment in time.

It was perfect. I had the skirt remade into a cape fit for a queen, or in this case a Zambian Chieftainess. I returned to the Mpongwe region and presented the royal garb and the tiara to her highness. Her smile spread from one ear to the other as she lifted the crown from its case and placed it on top of the pill box hat. She pulled my robe over her royal robe - adorning herself in layers of beauty. I smiled, letting it spread across my face too when I heard the Christmas music from eighth grade playing in my head and I remembered my own royal velvety skirt swaying as I moved across the floor to "Silver Bells."

As expected, the Chieftainess wanted photos taken of her in her new attire. The huge yard, with towering anthills in the background worked as a perfect backdrop to a most unlikely character.

She allowed the team to gather around her once her initial portraits were taken and each image on the camera accurately recorded this unique moment in our lives. The only problem we had from this experience was that she now wanted our camera as a gift. Dr. Henry, I learned, was most gracious and generous with his possessions. He freely and without hesitation handed over the small camera that once hung from the small black case on his belt. It seemed like a reasonable gift in exchange for our visit and our permission to leave her royal palace intact and alive.

We gave our compliments to her and acknowledged the guards that flanked her, standing erect in their too-large clothing. We left just before nightfall down the dusty road to exit her property. Slowly she disappeared from the rear view mirror - framed by the gigantic ant hills and bronzed huts, standing wrapped in retro velvet and adorned with bridal crystals that reflected in the African sun. She was the ebony queen in many ways, ruler of the vast tribal land, and stood second to none.

Royalty is present in the tribal regions - all seventy-two of them. On the other end of royalty, like any other country in the world, live the extreme poor, struggling for existence. That is where I wanted to go; to meet those who needed our help.

As I was packing the day before my departure for this trip to Africa, our church in Ohio mailed a box of bandages, ointments, aspirin, and an envelope with handwriting on the outside that said, "It is not much, but it is all that I have. Please give this to the poor in Africa." The contents of the unnamed envelope consisted of coins and two bills totaling $4.00. I put the envelope in my carry-on and hoped that we could do something with it for someone.

The following day, after our visit to the chief, we took a walk with the director from Campus Crusade through the compound of Chifubu, a dense deposit of the most impoverished people in the Copperbelt region of Zambia. Dirt homes, strengthened with mud and topped with thatched elephant grass roofs lined the narrow dirt path that meandered through the structures. Unemployment and illness was the commonality of the people. In monetary terms, they were poor, but rich in their faith. *How ironic,* I thought. The U.S. is rich monetarily, and often poor in their faith. *Who was more blessed,* I wondered.

I asked to go into one of the homes as we walked through the village. There was a wooden fence about five feet high made of split logs, uneven and gaping in most areas. The house's security - twine draped over the adjacent post. Wild dogs were often seen running in the street.

We entered the dirt yard and a woman emerged from the shack with a rag tied securely over her unkempt hair, and another cloth secured around her waist to keep the red dirt from her labor from staining her worn dress. Five tiny children hung around from her knees in heights from her calf to her waist, like a flight of stairs. No one had shoes.

Smoke from an open fire rose from a small cast iron pot in the corner of the yard. Beans were the dinner for the day, and there didn't look like enough to provide for everyone.

"She is a widow, and these are her children," our guide explained. She represented the majority of the families here, either widowed, or abandoned by husbands who left their responsibilities as fathers and husbands turning to alcohol or other women.

"What does she need?" I asked, wanting to help this woman and her children.

"She needs money for rent, and beans for the month," the translator said.

"How much would that be?" I asked, and started to mentally add up the amount of kwatcha that I had in my backpack, hoping that I had enough to provide for this struggling family of six.

"16,800 kwatcha."

"Help me to calculate how much that is please," I requested.

"That is $4. She needs $3.00 for rent, and $1.00 for a bag of beans."

The envelope from the anonymous donor from Ohio came immediately to mind. "We can do that," I said, a lump forming in my throat. *God has provided for this widow and her children*, I thought.

I enjoyed wholeheartedly handing the money over to the woman and it was visible without a doubt that she loved it more than I. The extreme gratitude that had overwhelmed her, brought tears to my eyes. Her face, and those of the children were etched in my mind like a photo.

The following year, our medical team was working in an abandoned school building not far from Chifubu; the people came, desperate for medical care as there was none in the area, and no money for them to travel elsewhere.

Our team set up the clinic in the modest building treating over 300 patients that day, many of them were children. My place for that day was at the main pharmacy table dispensing medications that the physicians just a few feet away from me had prescribed for each illness.

Even though we worked fast and efficiently, two RNs could barely keep up with the demands of the multiple prescriptions.

I felt a tug of my sleeve as I was intensely counting out antibiotics for a child with pneumonia and looked up to see a woman, dressed in a clean street dress, with a child, clean and neat at her side.

"Do you remember me?" she asked.

I looked at her and her child and strained to think of where I would have met her. How would I have known this fairly well-dressed women and her child?

"I am the lady who you visited last year. You gave me money for rent and beans for me and my children," she said.

The $4.00 lady! I thought.

"I most certainly *do* remember you...but you look so different!" I said. "You look wonderful! What has happened to you?"

"After you left last year, I went and asked at the school who you were and why would a stranger come and give me money.

"They told me that you were a Christian woman from the U.S. and was the president of OMNI," She continued. "I asked them if I could volunteer at the school hoping that someday you and your team would return, so that I could thank you.

"After volunteering for several months, they gave me a job and the money that I make provides food and rent for my family...no one had ever done anything like that before for me." Tears freely fell from her cheeks.

I was amazed that the money I gave her had provided her with so much hope and initiative. I asked her to come over to the side of the building near our tables - out of eyesight. "Use this for your children and keep doing what you are for them, I said, laying a few dollars into her hand. "I am so pleased to see what has happened to you." The small amount of money would hopefully buy more food.

The following year, our team was once again working out of the same school building, this time, now a functioning school thanks to the many donors from the U.S. who had faith in OMNI to provide for the poor children of Chifubu. My eyes kept scanning the room for Phoebe to return again this year. The church in Ohio had sent money for her and her family as the news of the $4 lady had spread to a now amazing story of God's provisions.

Phoebe returned and she and her children were surviving and thriving on her small income. Not all needs were met, however, such as school and clothing, so the money that I had for her would be essential for these needs. "Come here and sit down with me," I said. "I have something for you." I took her hand. People watched us now and my fear for her grew. I didn't want to make her a target - best to hand her money in private.

I pulled a petite bible from my backpack - money was hidden between the thin pages of the precious little book. I laid it in her trembling hands.

"God has been watching over you and continues to bless you and your family," I said.

She took the bible and tucked it into her skirt and left with her children. She smiled as she turned back just before leaving the room.

The following year, our clinic was held at the same location, treating the same mass of impoverished people. The numbers grew to over 400 this year and the school had over forty students who were being educated.

Phoebe never showed. I feared for the worse and finally, at the end of the day, asked about her and her family.

"She moved to Lusaka - the capital," explained the school organizer.

"She is now a seminary student in the school of divinity," she said with a smile. "She is going to be a pastor someday!"

Our $4 lady was a miracle in the making. My heart pounded with pure joy and pride. I couldn't have been any happier for her. Apparently, Phoebe used the small support that she had been given and with her own efforts and courage turned her life around. The dramatic turn would also benefit her children who otherwise would have succumbed to extreme poverty as well. It was the best $4 ever spent.

An equally as impoverished compound within the city, but far more dangerous, was that of Kawama. Our team was invited there to run a medical clinic in the building of an existing government clinic who had no supplies and only a few analgesics in their undersized pharmacy. The needs in this densely populated inner city shanty town was staggering.

The staff, all dressed in beautiful white starched uniforms, agreed to help us with registering patients and to assist with interpretation, as few here could speak English.

The pediatrician had no separate room to work in, so he set up a table in the hallway. Dr. Henry had the back room to do exams and for me to set up the pharmacy. We had another physician who was off somewhere at a meeting of officials, so he didn't get a separate space, and my son Mark took photos.

The lines were endless and the patients we treated were being diagnosed with multiple diseases - HIV/AIDs, TB, and leprosy seemed to be bundled diagnoses for many of the young men who came in.

Dr. Henry examined a young man who had pus seeping from the base of his fingernails as well as multiple small lesions on the rim of his upper ear. "Leprosy," Dr. Henry said to me. "He also has STD and needs antibiotics."

As quick as I could, I filled syringes with penicillin and antibiotics for the STD. The boy would have to go to the HIV clinic for long term follow up.

Mark entered the back room looking pale and sweaty. He laid on the only gurney that we had in the tiny room. I immediately put my hand on his forehead - cold and clammy. I kept an eye on him and gave him water as I continued to fill the syringes. My only nurse also became ill and, she too, fell into one the chairs, slumping over.

Dr. Henry and I worked together well, which was a great thing, as we now had to step up our pace. Four men were now sitting on a wooden bench, pants unzipped, and each ready for their injections.

I stared at the left side of the bench, and gave the 2cc injections in the left hip, and then the right hip of the first man, and went down the row from there until, I had completed all eight doses of penicillin. Through the interpreter we told the men that the women that they had been in intimate contact with were most likely also infected and needed to come to our clinic for treatment. It was unlikely that many of them would comply. It was our responsibility, however, to educate them and make the attempt to reach their partners for evaluation.

Dr. Henry continued to see more patients and I ended up doing lab tests, running the pharmacy, and helping him any way I could. I kept Mark within ear and eye-shot.

Around one, the nurse in the white uniform from up front, walked through with a white duck under her arms down the hall and to the back of the building. *Strange*, I thought but later learned that the duck did not survive - he became lunch for their staff.

Our team had water and a granola bar and kept on working.

At the end of the day, we were exhausted but felt that we had effectively treated some of the most critical patients in this area. Mark felt better and was able to walk out on his own. We had used up our entire malaria and HIV test kits and had run out of penicillin.

It had been a great hard working day and at the end, we thanked the in country staff for their assistance and hospitality. We all gathered outside the blue painted building to take a photo before we boarded our bus to leave. The wooden gates were now locked around the clinic soon came to a close. Tomorrow would be another day at the clinic, and then we would make the twenty-three hour flight back to the U.S.

"B" is for Business and Burgundy

Purchasing a vehicle in a foreign country has proven to be an interesting experience for me and our organization. We found that with the work that we did, a vehicle was essential not only when we were in the country, but for our staff to provide necessary care, food and supplies for the children that we served.

The newspapers are limited and show cars, trucks, and various vehicles of transportation for sale. One does not know if the vehicle is sound, or has legitimate odometer readings. After a great deal of searching the papers and using the Internet for imported cars from Japan, I was instructed to try a new route.

Roughly twelve vehicles sat in a small lot next to the only grocery store in town. There were trucks, cars, and SUVs of all colors, years, and conditions. I was told that I could purchase a car from this lot, pay cash, and leave with a "new to me" vehicle. I was prepared as much as I could, with some cash, and courage.

We drove up to the lot and Felton got out, instructing me to stay in the rented vehicle so that my presence would not inflate the going price. I watched Felton run through the lot, looking at only three vehicles from the twelve that would suffice for our needs.

He came back with the following: "We can get the burgundy car now for cash. The body looks good, and the interior is even better. I say we go for it."

New to this experience, we had several questions and answers that went back and forth before I agreed to the purchase.

"I'll be right back," he said as he ran from the car to the owner of the lot.

Within minutes, an extremely short man climbed into our back seat alongside me and began to tell me of the terms of the sale. Through the interpretation and help of Felton we agreed on the terms of the sale in cash. Cash counted out first by me, then Felton, then by the man in the back seat. Once the amount was confirmed the currency was exchanged and I signed the sale of agreement, then he was gone - just like that.

I sat there and watched this little man and his friend run down the street with our money, and finally disappeared into the distance.

"What have we done?" I asked Felton.

"Not to worry, he has run to the city hall to prepare the documents and will be right back," Felton tried to assure me.

It seemed more than risky and absolutely out of a movie to be honest, but there we were in the middle of this situation.

About an hour later, the man came running down the street with papers in his hand and documents for me to sign.

Again, the back seat of our car was the office and we signed all papers and were handed the key to our new, used burgundy car. From this point forward, the car would soon get another name, not out of adoration, but frustration.

Traveling to the country on business periodically has to happen to keep an organization intact. Being there is necessary to keep the mission going, and to keep the mice from playing or carrying away the cheese completely.

In our early years, I ran an informative meeting for potential medical team members. It was there that I met Dr. Jim. As I remember, he arrived late, sat in the back row and appeared to be quite uninterested. A tall man with broad shoulders, a handsome face, and a strong jaw; he was impressive. As a surgeon, he was used to asking for what he needed and getting it, and checking off things in life that did not suit him. He also had a list of adventures that he wanted to experience. I found out quickly that going to Africa was on his so called bucket list. From his demeanor, and his lack of interest in the details, I thought that this informative meeting about a mission in Africa would not be his cup of tea.

The first meeting described the mission of OMNI, the dates that we would travel, how the clinics worked, and what was required of you should you choose to serve on the team. Attend and you would hear the stats of Africa, why OMNI was in Zambia, what was involved, your cost to be on the team...and so on. About twelve people showed up. Some wanted to hear what it might be like if they inserted themselves into a dream of going to Africa. Immunizations, travel, security risks, lack of lodging, etc. I could see the glaze rise in the eyes of those people who thought they were in way over their heads. Telling a group about the many adventures of going to Africa was exciting. The tale would well be worth telling!

To my surprise Jim showed up for the next meeting. He and several other souls seeking either adventure or service joined the team. It was interesting and at time revealing to see the different personalities prepare themselves for the travel to Africa. Despite all of the information and preparation that I could instill, each person harbored an image of what Africa would be and what he or she would become in Africa. Some envisioned game parks, safaris, and khaki-colored clothes. Others could see themselves playing primitive drums in distant villages and somehow fitting into the culture. I looked for those who truly wanted to serve the extreme poor and kept my internal radar on for those who could be a potential problem on any team, especially this one.

During our final meeting we discussed how we packed the medical supplies and medications - each bag strategically color coded for easy identification. White duct tape indicated non-medical items such as clothing, shoes, or school supplies that would be given to the children in local the schools. Green tape indicated that the contents were medical in nature. These bags would contain bandages, syringes, ace wraps, stethoscopes, and various items needed in a mobile clinic. The bags donned with red tape contained medications used in our pharmacy including analgesics, antibiotics, and ointments for wounds, eye and ear washes, and baby formula. All medications had to be meticulously listed on the manifest and would include the amount of the medication, the expiration dates and the dosages of each drug. No bags could contain narcotics, or controlled substances used here in the U.S.

Each team member has to pack their own carry-on and only the travel boots can go into a team duffle to allow all available space to go toward the medical supplies. This formula creates some interesting packing challenges, given the small bag has to carry enough clothes and toiletries for the entire two weeks.

Jim packed his alligator loafers as he learned that we would be staying in a lodge. *Safari* is probably the word that came to his mind along with imagining fine South African wines sure to be served on the veranda of our *Out of Africa* estate.

Silly man, I thought. I warned him that the loafers were not necessary; the lodge was not what he was thinking it to be. I told him that the huts have dirt floors and there isn't any electricity until we got into town, which would be several days later. There, we would have a basic hotel - and electricity was not guaranteed.

I packed his fancy shoes anyway, smiling as I zipped them into a gallon plastic bag then into the corner of the duffle near the spam and toilet paper.

We traveled for fifty-two grueling hours via Nairobi, Kenya, sleeping on hard tables in the tiny coffee shop at the end of the small, hot airport in our twelve-hour layover. The place was pretty empty, except for a few wooden tables with benches - our respite stop before traveling on. Heads lowered to tables and some rested against the wall taking comfort on the floor. We took off almost a half day later for our destination. After a short flight we landed in Malawi, only to let some passengers off and on.

From the rear opening of the plane the airport and the many rows of green, lush fields of maize caught my attention - Iowa Fair winners no doubt. As the back hatch opened to let in some air, I got up to stretch my legs and take a quick picture of the emerald colored fields of Malawi.

"No pictures allowed!" someone yelled. "We will confiscate your camera if you do that again."

I sat down quickly. *Not a problem*, I thought as I tucked the camera in my backpack. The picture was now imbedded in my mind anyway. It was beautiful, small, and inaccessible land mass rich in soil and rich in intrigue.

A few passengers toting carry-ons entered the plane and took only few minutes to get situated. Each person had clothing that represented their tribal heritage. Some wore suits, but all were privileged according to the norms of this part of the world.

I flew through there years later on my way back from Nairobi with the body of a government official who had been gunned down in the city. All safety precautions were reviewed and all passengers were required to be securely fastened into their seats. In preparation for landing in the capital of Zambia on that trip, the air space was cleared for landing. We had dignitaries, sitting in the first few rows of first class, who accompanied the body home. One never knows who you travel with, or what has gone on before your departure.

Landing in Lusaka, with Jim and the team, was like a homecoming for me. I knew what to expect and was prepared and ready to accept the adventure on this trip. We had to pass through customs, come out of the airport, find the driver, and secure what we could for the next part of our journey. Customs can take an enormous amount of time depending on who is on the other side of the counter. There are those that want to examine every single item and question its purpose and validity; others open the bags, look quickly through the middle, and sometimes the corners, and wave you on through. This particular time, we had every bag searched and every item removed. We were fortunate that this particular time, only a few medications were confiscated. Prenatal vitamins this month was illegal and all were taken. My gut told me that they were sold within hours of us leaving. We only hoped that eventually, someone would benefit from the dietary enhancement of the vitamins.

A large bus was our vehicle this time around - perfect for pulling an open trailer of duffel bags. We drove ten hours north, broke down only once, and arrived safely. I thought it was a good trip!

The team traveled to the deep bush and stayed in Agape, the village in the tribal region under the local Chieftainess. We arrived around midnight, and after three days of travel with no sleep, personalities that were once polished, became tarnished with raw emotions. Our clothes smelled of dirt and sweat and so did we. We all looked like we had been dragged in by the cat. We descended from the bus to be met by complete darkness, tribal men with torches, and no amenities of the lodge dreamt about throughout the trip.

"Where the hell have you taken me, Karen?" Jim asked. He looked exhausted and out of his element. I wasn't sure if he was angry or frightened or both. Nonetheless, it clearly was a question that he wanted answered and it appeared that he expected that I would have the answer.

"We are here, Jim! I said with utter excitement to be back in the deep bush. "It's a lot to take in. You will be fine in the morning. Our hut is over there and once the sun comes up, you will see what I was telling you about." I didn't understand the grumbled words that came from his mouth after that, and frankly didn't care. I was back home in the deep bush of Africa, bordering the great Savanna. I could not help but smile about his alligator shoes located next to the toilet paper and spam in the team duffel.

We unloaded in the dark. First thing I hoped to find was my flashlight.

Jim survived the trip and actually said that he grew as a person and as a physician. He seemed to enjoy getting back to the basics of life, caring for tribal members with little or no medical amenities and almost no paperwork. He seemed to smile more and complain less. He went home after that trip and according to his family the change in him was a good thing to see.

As the years go by, I am convinced that nothing good happens in Kabwe.

Traveling to the country on business periodically has to happen in order to keep an organization intact. Being there is necessary to keep the mission going, and to keep the mice from playing or carrying away the cheese completely.

As president of OMNI, I had a large building project to organize. Dr. Jim was now our VP, and Africa had changed him a great deal as a man, and created a more empathetic physician. Even his wife and children commented on how Africa had changed Jim for the better. It also changed how he packed. He never took his alligator shoes again.

I needed to travel there during the off season with the medical team to move the vision and the projects on the ground in a positive way. Taking care of business from 3,000 miles away via Internet, when few people can access it even in the second largest city in Zambia, is a monumental challenge.

Seven hours later, we landed in the capital. Business was on the agenda. Customs was always a challenge. Purchase a visa upon entry, having the right denomination in currency, fill out the lengthy white paper of visa entry form. The paper had been photocopied many times, and was cut in half by hand to save paper. Despite the basic supplies in the airport for visa entry, all documentation was scrutinized and double checked for authenticity.

Check the following:

- Name as it appears on your passport. Check
- Passport number and issue date: Check
- Birth date and address in your country of origin. Check
- Address of your stay while in Zambia. Check
- How many days will you stay? Check. Miss one day and you are in violation.
- State the purpose of your visit. Business or vacation? "B". Check.

We arrived in our team shirts, white for business, made it through the customs line, got our four duffels and met our staff director on the other side of the customs wall. There was a cluster of men waiting there with signs to identify themselves as drivers, or representatives for a waiting organization. Each would guide you safely to your destination.

Felton was there with no sign of identification or poster to catch our attention, as I knew him well. He had worked for me for several years in as our country director for our projects on the ground and for our school. As soon as he spotted me, he smiled - almost giggling. After loading into the car he had waiting for us, we gassed up and headed into the country. Upon arrival we exchanged a few U.S. dollars for enough kwatcha to purchase gas and some food along our route. Details were well-planned on our end, however, things were not always well-planned in the country of arrival.

I smiled as I looked around the car Felton had picked us up in - it was the new used car that we had recently found on the Internet and had it shipped from Japan for our use. How wonderful to see the car. I had wired money over to Africa for the purchase of a car so that our director could use it daily for bringing children to and from the OMNI site, driving to the city market, and purchasing over 400 pounds of food for the children each month. It was a lovely burgundy color Land Rover and was the first OMNI car in Zambia. I could tell Felton was very proud to be allowed to drive it, as he grinned from ear to ear as he drove.

In preparation for our arrival, I had asked that Felton purchase and install the best security system that he could find for the vehicle. He went to several auto shops in the city and had a unique system installed that took a puzzle master to figure it out to start the car - you basically had to reach under the dash, like using braille, to find the button. Push the button at the same time that you turn the ignition. Once the car turns over, quickly push another button on the key fob to secure yourself in the vehicle. All doors and windows now should be locked, and you in it as well. To get out of the vehicle, you had to reverse the process in the same sequence or an alarm would go off and you could be arrested for being stuck in your own vehicle!

It was ingenious, as far as alarms go in Africa. We had a secure car when parked and locked, and we were in a secure vehicle when in the same car in motion. I loved it.

We left the airport in Lusaka, traveling about 1,000-feet before our first checkpoint for the airport security. The armed guard glanced into our car, looked Jim and I over then our driver. We passed the test and he moved us on. Only three more checkpoints to go and a hard seven-hour drive.

The poorly graded dirt road, mostly red in color and heavy with traffic, was an adventure in itself. Approaching us were busses clearly overloaded with Zambian nationals, luggage strapped to the roof, bundles of homemade luggage bursting from the tight spaces of this worn, open air, form of public transportation. Air within the vehicles despite windows being open is dense, reeking of body odor, and African soil. Chickens bound at their skinny ankles accompanied some families, presumably, that evening's dinner. Oxen carts came in the other direction keeping to the side so that vehicles could pass. Trucks, rolled down that turbulent road with open beds carrying goats and pigs. More trucks passed with families on the back, children riding with no seat belts, mothers with babies, piled on top of heaps of ground maize. All had an awareness that this was the best that they could do short of walking for days.

The countryside was lined with miles of open space filled with kops of trees that had been shaped and painted into the African horizon. There were no street signs or lights to guide your travel. No speed limit which allows truckers and independent cars of means to travel at excessive speeds, leaving a trail of dust, people scattering, and any animal in its path, left as a mark in the long road north.

Our first checkpoint on the road north was met by a national MP, armed with an AK47. He looked at our vehicle, circled it, then checked the sticker on the front left corner of the windshield showing our registration in the country. Again, after looking into the car from the driver side window and seeing two Americans in team shirts, and our driver, all looking in order, we were motioned to pass with a wave of his hand. As I turned back to look, he walked back into the half overseas container parked on the side of the road that functioned as his office.

Semi-trucks were not so fortunate to pass. Multiple trucks had been pulled over for inspection, obviously not passing and being detained for reasons unknown to us. Foster explained that the trucks were coming south from the Congo on this road and were being inspected for illegal contents such as ivory, human trafficking and drugs.

Despite traveling north against the flow, Kabwe was a different story that went south pretty fast...

With Felton at the wheel and Jim and I in the car, having just arrived, the officer on the side of the road in full uniform motioned for us to pull over as this was our second checkpoint. Every car was stopped, and every passport was being checked. Trucks, cars or various makes and conditions were all halted and ushered to the dirt pull over lane. I was hoping for a quick check and a release as we had many hours yet to travel on this already two-day journey.

Felton and I handed our passports to the officer and Jim followed from behind me in the back seat, offering his document of identity as well. The passports were examined page by page, and reviewed several times, and not returned as previously done at that last stop. The officer motioned for another colleague to join him at our window and a discussion ensued over our confiscated passports.

My passport was returned along with Felton; however, Jim's remained in the grasp of the police. Seconds passed as he looked in our car then at each one of us. "You are under arrest" he said to Jim. "Please get out of the car and come to my office." Jim reluctantly complied, being persuaded by the gun and the tone of the command.

"It appears that you have violated your visa." We were all motioned to get out of our car and stand by the officer. The madam here is clearly here on business as marked by the "B" on her passport, and her team shirt." You, sir, have a "V" on your visa indicating that you are here as a visitor, yet you wear the same team shirt."

A conversation that ensued in the tribal language between Felton and the officer got us nowhere it seemed from my observation. As the communication process seemed to increase in speed and intensity, the next English phrase was quite clear. Felton had just been arrested as well, for obstructing justice and both were to be taken into custody.

Felton told me to get back into our car and wait while he straightened this situation out. I would have been happy to retreat, however, the car door was now locked. "Felton, just open it and I will get in and wait," I said.

His fumbling of the alarm button on the key ring clearly indicated a malfunction in the lock system. We were locked out, and my two guys were under arrest. Felton gave me his phone with the number of the U.S. Embassy pulled up for auto-dialing. When someone picked up on the other end, I quickly stated my name, and began to repeat the phone number that I was calling from.

Perfect timing, I thought as the embassy was about to close for the day. What was not as successful was the sound of the phone going dead as minutes ran out of the phone. I only had three digits more to recite of his number to the embassy. Close, but that only works in horseshoes and doesn't count. I handed the phone back to Felton and we both felt our hearts sink to our stomachs.

Felton, now being somewhat flustered with the whole situation began to argue with the officer who was detaining Jim. Voices escalated until it was clear that another step in the wrong direction for us had occurred. I could see them walk away, fading into the distant group of small buildings near the roadside. They disappeared as they entered the metal overseas container that was the police office for this location.

This scene wasn't looking good from my perspective. It was getting near dusk, and we had been detained for over thirty minutes at this point.

I could hear Jim repeat over and over that we had no money to pay the fine, whatever that was. My heart began to pound as I listened to their conversation, feeling more than conspicuous as my skirt was hanging heavily with over $20,000 of $100 dollar bills pinned under it in various locations from the waist to the hem. I brought money in to pay our project expenses and felt like the Bank of Barclay at that point. We had not opened a bank account of our own and were dealing with all payments in cash. Hard to believe, but we were on the learning curve that was headed straight up.

We had taken a stand over the years to at no cost or circumstance would we pay off a bribe or a threat. We were not going to fall into that now, however, I questioned if that was prudent right about now.

We stuck to our plan of no payoffs. Trucks with chickens and goats came and went, as I stood by myself near the locked car on the side of the road in the not-so-friendly village of Kabwe at sundown. Mothers with babies, men and small children were allowed to come and go. It was dark and I didn't feel like this was going well. My skirt hung low to the ground as the wind picked up.

Illuminated by the headlight of a detained truck, I could see Felton and Jim, walking back to me. *Thank God*, I thought. I had promised Jim's wife I wouldn't leave him in Africa. It was a scenario, that while standing there alone, I practiced making the call to her processing what words could describe Jim's detainment and eventual loss to an African prison. No matter what words I put together, or tried to make it sound better than it was, my conversation in my head remained dire.

As they got within the shadows, I could see that they both seemed to be smiling. The stars were starting to come out and maybe our luck had changed. Large overstuffed trucks and busses were still held at ransom on both sides of the road. People and small livestock were all around us, stuck, and held at bay. I was getting chilled from the evening wind and the fear of being left alone.

"What happened?" I asked with great curiosity and extreme relief.

"I had to give a gift from my heart," Jim replied. He paused and smiled again.

"And what gift from your heart did you give?" I looked at him relieved, yet surprised that he was as calm as he appeared.

He opened his wallet to show that it was now empty. The gift was in the form of a $100 U.S. bill, the only bill that he had placed there, with the remaining bills hid in a waist pouch. I was convinced that this was a bargain compared to the currency that remained under my skirt.

Both men were released to me, or so it seemed. We were all free, but stranded without entrance into our car, and it was now pitch dark out. At least I had company again other than the trucks filled with livestock and weary, detained nationals.

Felton was quite resourceful, and told Jim and I to wait outside the car. "Great I thought, left alone again in Kabwe." We had no other choice but to wait since all doors remained locked. He came back thankfully after a few minutes, which seemed much longer. Jim and I agreed that we were very fortunate to even be there together and released from confinement.

Jim was still giving some details of his arrest. He told me about how the police said he would love the food, bread and water, and that he would have a nice cot to sleep on. Jim was clearly rattled and I suspected that he was thinking of his home back in the states and wondered once again. "Where the hell have you taken me, Karen?" I did not want to respond to his obvious fears as I really felt we could get out of this one. At least I hoped so.

Felton showed up with minutes loaded on his cell phone from "a brother" somewhere out there in the dark of night who loaned him a phone. There were a few small block dirt buildings that I could see when the sun was up earlier that day, however, looked nothing like it resembled a storefront for cell phone business.

"We are back in business," Felton said.

I thought, *And, what business is that since we are still here and stranded?*

He called the owner of the auto shop in Ndola, and of course, he was not in. It was past closing time. From that attempt he called his wife to explain the dilemma we were in. She had no car, but was willing to run across town at night upon Felton's request and go to the owner of the garage and have him phone us with the code to open the car.

Jim leaned over to me and made the snide comment, "This doesn't happen at home, you know."

"You are most correct. It does not, but aren't you having fun, Jim? I know that you can do this!" I felt like a cheerleader, after the team had just lost the big game.

We could hear a lot of conversation, that was rapid and in the tribal language. "OK, OK!" he said. Felton pushed some buttons on the door handle and once in the car, pushed another button that was hid under the steering wheel that disarmed the locking system. We all got back into the car, with Jim in the front next to Felton, and me in the back, with my heavy skirt.

Now, we had mastered the coveted code for the new lock and could operate the burgundy car. We were on our way! Revised ETA: 3 am.

We had traveled this dangerous road the year before with a full team, packed into a bus, pulling a small trailer. I was destined as they say to ride in the presidential car with Felton and drill him for information about our project and what was new on the ground here in Africa.

Our job was to follow the bus, and make sure that they arrived ahead of us even if it was only by a few minutes. After all, we had the cell phone, the minutes, and the money.

We stopped at the second small town along the road north to Ndola. There was little there other than a few local pubs, vegetable stands, an auto chop shop, and a large population of unemployed random people looking for a few ways to make the next Kwatcha enabling them to buy local brew.

Most everyone on the bus had to use the restroom, of which we had to supply. We pulled up to an abandoned lot enclosed by metal gates that were worn and borrowed from another site. The path to the small building in the back was a small dirt dog path, laden with litter and thugs from the town. When we approached the building, there was a man outside collecting funds and handing out five squares of toilet paper with each purchase to use the restroom. It was worth the equivalent of six cents to use the facility even if there was no running water and the sinks were broken. Relief comes at a price - even here. Great care was taken so those who were new to foreign travel did not wander off or make conversation with the local entrepreneurs.

Following the bus for the first four hours was uneventful until we passed the second checkpoint and we were several kilometers north. We were in the middle of a vast dark uninhabited rural area marked randomly by small dirt paths into the bush. Some were preceded by stones piled about knee high or higher to signal that local brew could be had in this direction. Sparks flew from the trailer's left rear tire, and within seconds the tire flew off and into the elephant grass that paralleled the road. The back corner of the trailer fell to the pavement with more sparks causing the bus driver to slow down and quickly pull to the side of the road. We were following the fireworks of a breakdown and it was not the fourth of July.

The wheel and tire were gone, the back of the trailer was damaged, and we were going to have to unload everything and everybody. Sixteen tired team members filed off the bus into the dark, cold ditch. There are no streetlights in the deep countryside of Africa and no AAA services. Our only chance of getting to our destination was to unload all duffels and wedge them among the team.

This decision did not come immediately, as there were many plans that were tossed back and forth, none of them viable solutions to this magnitude of a problem. Our guard walked around the bus with his AK47 slung over his shoulder. Our team huddled together as the night was cold with a slight wind. One of the ladies on our team had a small guitar and decided that music and songs would help the moral. We sat in the ditch in pitch dark singing. It actually was an unexpected blessing in disguise.

As we sang, the driver and some of the men off-loaded the trailer and loaded the bus to the ceiling with twenty-nine duffels filled with medical supplies. The remaining seven duffels had to be fit into the burgundy car, making both vehicles stuffed. There were small spaces near the ceiling of the bus that we could slide some of the younger team members in, similar to the last layer of a sardine can before it is closed.

The trailer had to be left behind, however, leaving it would surely set us up for theft. The driver's mechanic was left to guard the broken down trailer, and was outfitted with a blanket, some trail bars, water in a jug, and matches to make a fire. Someone would be back for him tomorrow. I think he drew the short straw on this assignment.

It was another late ETA. We arrived at the campsite to start our first clinic at four in the morning.

Tired and a bit disoriented, we all managed to set up the clinic under the canopy of the trees near the Agape Village deep in the bush. It was typical to have over 300 people show up for medical care in one day - a number that over the years would double and even exceed to 700 a day. All people were seen, treated, and cared for. Our team worked like a mash unit, and methodically and compassionately cared for the poor.

Joshua showed up once again at the clinic. He looked well and nourished. This time he wanted to go to school. He was persistent and I had to appreciate his drive to be educated. He would argue and plead his case until he got what he wanted - often times exhausting me. I agreed to pay for tuition to go to a private school deep within the bush, where he would be a resident and get an education, food, and perhaps a future. The school enrolled about 400 students and was funded by a church in Great Britain. His tuition was paid directly to the school and the reports of his accomplishments and activities were sent to me directly. He did well and was a good student. On breaks, he would walk several miles home to his village to see his mother. He was absorbing the blessings and gifts given to him.

Wound care was tended to as though in the battlefields of poverty with life depended on it. Miracles were happening with each cleansing and bandaging of the wounds. Infected ear drums, pneumonias, and malaria cured with medications. Few people in the bush had HIV/AIDS, but the numbers continued to rise over the years as more and more people managed to walk or travel into town on a bicycle, and become infected through unprotected sex. Condoms were not available and if they were, not many would purchase them due to lack of funds. The other problem was that they were used over and over until they were torn. The people lived off the land. They didn't think much about medical care or prevention - it just wasn't obtainable. Our clinics provided the only care for these people once a year. Yet, in the one-time encounter, people's lives were being saved and souls were being reached.

Land of Our Own

Each time we went back to the states, we brought back pictures of our work with the people and stories that encouraged others to support the work that we were doing in Africa. OMNI team members continued to give presentations in churches, schools, Rotary Clubs, and in private homes. Never was money asked for but each talk inspired others to support the poor through our work. OMNI became the vehicle of which others could make a difference in the lives of orphans and the poor in Africa and have accountability for every dollar.

OMNI eventually raised enough funds to purchase a small farm north of the copper mines near Kitwe. The area was rich farmland and the property seemed perfect to start an orphanage. A long driveway lead to a small ranch style home, previously owned by an elderly couple moved in with their adult children. The twelve-acres was more than they could continue to manage but it was perfect for us.

Mango, coffee, popo, and bananas grew to the north of the house. A large ant hill, covered now in grass, stood just beyond the home. Just over the crest of the hill, was a beautiful stream that bordered the property. In the front five-acres stood two dilapidated buildings that once housed horses - complete with remnants of the stalls and the grooming area. Horses had not occupied this building in over a decade and the roof and walls were mostly gone. The foundation lent itself to our imaginations and we envisioned the future site of a beautiful building that would soon be home to orphaned children.

We purchased the farm with a cash sale, and actually found the price to be quite low for the property. We had a building team come from the states and worked on renovations of the house, paint, and completed some yard clean up. The former horse stalls were measured and plans were drawn up for the new orphanage.

Felton and his wife moved into the house for security reasons, and to start planting crops that could sustain some of the children's needs and become self-sufficient. The first symptom of greed also started to grow; the portion of land that we allowed Felton to plant for his family was flourishing and the land prepared for OMNI crops was barely producing a productive crop. Felton was using our funds to keep his crops healthy and allowing little of the funds to be applied to OMNI's crops.

In all, this land designated for orphans seemed like a reasonable and viable plan. The only problem was that the children were not in this region. The homes in this area had once been owned by wealthy landowners, gentlemen farmers so to speak. It was not an area that was known to the poor.

The land was beautiful and would be suitable for a single family dwelling, but you would have to import children, bus them to a school and frankly, the idea wasn't working.

We realized our errors and now had property on our hands that needed to be sold. *Who in this country could afford this property?* I wondered. I feared that we were stuck and our money was held up in real-estate.

"Let's put an ad in the paper and see what happens," suggested Felton.

The idea seemed lame at best, but we had no other choice than to try it. In a worse-case scenario, we would be out the cost of the ad.

Within a week, we had a full price offer payable in cash from a man coming in from Australia who needed a home. We managed to make a small amount of profit from the sale and now had funds to find land that would be suitable for children in need.

Out of the Depths of Poverty

As fate would have it once again, we met a widow in town that came to the Campus Crusade for Christ's office while we were there delivering some supplies for their ministry. She taught school in an abandoned building and cared for children in a rural area of Ndola. Her husband, a local pastor had just died that year, and she carried out the work that the two of them had been doing as their ministry to the poor. HIV/AIDs had claimed his young life leaving her with four small children and now noticeably declining health.

"Please come to my home so that I can introduce you to my children and then we can go to the village where I teach the poor," she insisted. Her home was neat, and clean, small, and welcoming. In a shed attached to the tiny house were over fifty tiny chicks, peeping, and scratching for food. "I raise these chicks, and then sell them for a profit to feed my children. It's all that I have for income."

We gathered up her two smallest children and dropped them off at her sister's home just a few streets away from where she lived and drove the fifteen minutes out into the countryside to the village of George. There was a long dirt path that resembled the makings of a road, however, few cars traveled here since no one could afford one. There was no industry, or reason to go to George as it was an isolated farming community, with no stores except for a privately-owned local brew shack where meager profits from farming were being consumed in the form of wicked homemade alcohol sludge. It was the only thriving business in the village.

We made our way around the hand-planted corn fields, where women and men were toiling under the hot sun, grooming the fields with handmade hoes. The tools were made with local lumber to create the crude handle, and the blade was made of metal, and attached by driving the sharp end into the wood almost like a nail embedded in a board. Some of the older handles had tribal carvings near the metal blade creating a signature effect of ownership. Worn, sore hands had gripped the wood creating authentic grooves from hours of toil.

We came to a black metal gate, weather worn and lacking most of its original paint. It was the entrance to the community center of the village and housed a single cinder block building with two large rooms and a leaky tin roof. The paint on the building was probably, at one time, beautiful, and now had chipped and revealed layers of paint underneath that created the most gorgeous ocean teal color swirled with shades of white and gray. It was a backdrop that looked like it could be an abstract painting hanging in a museum.

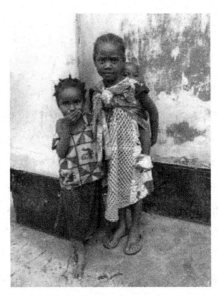

Children at George Compound

Inside the gate and immediately to the right in the corner sat a metal pump with a long handle, worn from years of attempts to draw water from the earth below. A small girl, barely high enough to extend her tiny arms, pumped the water. The life-saving water was the only source in the village and was contaminated by the cracked and exposed piping that penetrated the depth of the soil.

I watched as her tiny mouth opened to receive the water and her hands cupped the fluid as to catch anything that she could before it hit the ground around her bare feet.

People survived by coming to this well. Dishes were washed at this site and hands grasped the cold metal that brought the water from the earth.

The cement steps were broken and missing any full length of surface that was safe to walk on. We watched our footsteps carefully as we made our way into the building where you could hear a beautiful blend of small voices echoing in the barren room.

In front of a scratched, cracked chalkboard, stood a young man appearing no older than perhaps seventeen or eighteen. Across from him were about thirty children varying in ages from six to twelve. With a glance and a word, he commanded the children to stand, and be silent for the visitors. All dark brown eyes faced forward and watching as he instructed them to say "Hello" in unison in their tribal language. Barren dusty feet, stood on the cold cement floor, each pair remaining still with very few movements.

Teddy, young man from the village of George who had lived there since birth, had endured the poverty that the village endured. He appeared bright, spoke fluent English, and equally articulate in his own tribal language. He had impeccable manners and his natural command over the students was noticeable and admirable.

The pastor's wife introduced us to Teddy as her assistant teacher. In a short period of time, we found out that these children were from the most impoverished families, too poor to attend free government school.

"That doesn't make sense, if it is free, why can't they afford to go to school?" I asked.

"The government requires that you wear a uniform, which would cost about Kwatcha 90,000 ($12.00)," Teddy explained. The family did not have that money to provide for a uniform, so the children of these families would not be educated, and would live their lives in the village working in the fields like their parents and their parents before them. The village of George in an average home had no income as each household survived barely on subsistence farming. For the small minority, it was rare to find a job in town as a house servant, which paid around $50 per month. Walking the long distance to town which could be a four to five hour round trip was the price one had to pay for an income.

Teddy had grown up as a child from a poor family in George. He lived in the small community just outside of the city of Ndola and had managed to attend a school in a distant village. He was married, despite his young age, and had established a loving home for the two of them. He invited us to visit his home and lead our car down the dirt path as he walked in front of us to our destination.

Our vehicle meandered through the footpath to his home just a few minutes walking distance from the community building. The path was not intended for a vehicle and our tires drove over the rocks, earth, and the boundaries of the trail. We stopped in front of a little dirt house on the left. Teddy went into his home briefly and then emerged shortly after dressed in a clean shirt and pressed pants. I could see the pride and incredible sense of responsibility in him.

He came out of his home to properly greet us with a smile and a handshake that was most welcoming. From behind him came his wife, about nine months pregnant, legs and feet swollen beyond comfort. I looked down at her swollen ankles and the chickens that ran around them and realized that this young couple was about to give birth to a child with little modern medicine or amenities at their disposal. I admired them both. They were young, bright, engaged in the future, and trusting that God would provide.

Teddy wanted to be different and rise out of the downward spiral of poverty. He wanted to make a difference in his life and for the life of his family. He was giving back to his community with no pay, except the tremendous reward of seeing children learn and excel.

It was a moment in my life that I thought I had found not only the meaning to my life, but the meaning to sacrifice and dedication for others. This village is where OMNI should be and needs to be. This is where we can make a difference in the lives of children who want to learn but have no means. This is where we can bring medical care to those that have no care. It was our spot on earth to make OMNI happen. The smoke from the fires rose to the heavens.

Teddy was hired and continued to teach in the community building. There was no electricity, no restrooms except a couple of overused outhouses in the back of the building that serviced the entire community. Mothers of children stepped forward once Teddy asked for volunteers, and large cooking pots were brought to the site so that Nshima - the local food - could be prepared from the ground corn that OMNI purchased.

Two months into the school opening and the start of Teddy's career, the hands, feet and heart of the pastor's wife stopped as she lost her life from HIV/AIDS. Teddy had been handed the baton and was now leading the school. The next step was to bring in another teacher that could assist Teddy with the forty-seven students that showed up each day. Curriculum was developed, assignments given, and food was provided on a daily basis.

The OMNI School at George Village in Zambia, Africa was born.

Our time located at the small community building in George was deemed short as we knew that we could not be a free tenant for long. The community would use the building from time to time for meetings and gatherings of the elders and school would be disrupted to accommodate their schedules. Finding land of our own was essential to be able to house these needy children and provide a quality education and an atmosphere that was conducive to learning.

As prayers were answered, the Ndola City council donated sixty-acres of undeveloped land just outside the village. Initially they donated a smaller plot farther from the village, however, after a great deal of discernment and discussion, land portions were swapped with a motor cross organization. OMNI would receive a ninety-nine lease for seventeen hectors, in the middle of a vast area that was close to the village of George, an extremely impoverished farming community. The land was peppered with mango trees, ant hills, and brush. An ungraded dirt road ran through the parcel that cut the property diagonally in half and contained many footpaths that local villagers frequented. The land, according to many locals, had no value because of its location. The land was ours and valuable because we could serve the children and the poor that the country had not served.

The value to us was immeasurable. This was the new home of OMNI and our future school for children who had no access to education. It was the most beautiful site that I had ever imagined, and the vision was coming into focus. A beautiful earth colored rectangular shape stood out on the original title. When looking out across the undeveloped land, there wasn't much in the way of visually identifying marks except for a footpath headed that crossed over the property. Land became our roots in Zambia and the home for years to come.

A volunteer building team was assembled in the U.S. and within a few months traveled to Zambia to establish the beacons for the boundary of the property and demarcation of the school campus layout. Before any construction could be done, permits, stamps, and approvals had to come from the city council, ministry of education, and various powers that be to start the building process. We went from office to office, back again and then again the next day hoping to obtain a signature.

"He just left for lunch," was our reply in the first office.

"He left this morning for a funeral in the western region and will be back next week," came another response.

"The person that you need for this did not come in today and I don't have enough minutes on my phone to call him," said the last one.

Carbon paper was needed in another office and payments and stamps were needed down the hall. Each step was a painfully slow process, but within the week, our persistence paid off. We had the approval, and the required signatures to proceed with the project.

Rick our building director and I, along with Felton, now needed to rent a road grader to plow a new road and block off the old path that ran through our property. We went to several companies and found the equipment either too old to function, or the price was too high for us to manage it. The other challenge was to get the grader from its location of storage to the site. Transportation in a third world country is limited and resources to get large projects done are few. Rick did a fantastic job putting it all together and shortly after our departure, word came from Felton that the road had been completed and we now had access to the property.

The journey of a thousand steps had just begun. OMNI would make their identifiable footprint on the soil that God had provided for this ministry. OMNI had to raise the funds to build our own school and a cafeteria. Over the next two years, building continued creating two large structures that would house over one hundred children in grades one through seven. Feeding them every day was a necessity as the families that they lived with within the village had little to no food and each day was a struggle to provide one meal for the family. Children waited each night for a large pot of pumpkin leaves to boil over an open fire. This pot of leaf soup, with no other ingredients would be the meal for as many as ten people in the family. Everyone went to bed hungry hoping that the following day would provide a better meal.

OMNI provided nshima as the main dish of the noon meal; served on brightly colored plastic plates with small blue and red cups that held fresh milk. The paste-like food was made from corn and ground into a fine meal, then boiled in water for several minutes until a thick porridge substance was created. There is little nutritional value to this dish, however, because corn grows well here, it is the main staple for families.

Protein was essential for their growth, and we would send Felton into town each week to purchase 400 pounds of beans, dried fish called kapenta, onions, and tomatoes. This enhanced the nshima and is known as a "relish" to the local people.

Beans were considered a delicacy and not everyone could afford them. When beans were distributed to the poor by our team, every bean was precious and children and adults would kneel down in the grass to pick up any stray morsels that had accidently dropped and place them in their shetenges or pockets. Dirt made no difference in the desire for the beans.

Malsala Market was the people's market and the prices were as good as we could come by. Entering the open air market and seeing rows and rows of makeshift wooden booths manned by men and women selling their products, is a wondrous sight to see. A few items for purchase consisted of piles of dried beans, fish, vegetables, and meal, but you needed to know the language, and have a sense of security when you entered.

Felton took me into the market one afternoon and I trailed behind him keeping close as I was the only white woman in the entire bustling market and drew quite a stir among the locals. When they found out that I carried the money, I had many people ask for us to come and purchase from them. Purchasing large amounts could easily send the vendor home with enough money to take the next day off and maybe more. Most purchases were small and enough for a single family.

Dried beans were stacked in small mountainous shapes on top of handmade wooden tables. Some beans sat in mounds on the ground on a ragged plastic tarp.

"We don't buy from this one, and that one's prices are too high, "Felton would say to educate me on market purchases. "This one has rotten beans and I don't trust her," he explained as we hustled along the dense market, lined with vendors selling eggs, vegetables, and dried fish that smelled like river water.

We made our way along the dirt paths until we came to two women standing near their small bean stand.

"Oh, my brother, you are back and you brought a friend, I see," said the shorter woman.

"This is the president - my boss," Felton said, stepping back as he looked at me. "She runs the new school that we are building where all of the children eat their meals."

Handshakes, proper curtsies, and greetings were exchanged before Felton started to examine the beans.

"Ok," he said. "I want 400 kilograms of beans, divided into four bags."

We were motioned to follow the two women through a maze of small vendor stations, each watching as the white woman followed close behind, yelling for us to stop and buy whatever they were selling. A large sale had just been negotiated and everyone wanted to be in on the deal.

After going through rows of vendors, who were women selling their food supply from local fields and streams, some with babies on their backs, we arrived at a large wooden structure with a tarp nailed over the opening of the door. The boards were uneven and you could see daylight seeping in through the cracks providing very small amounts of light into the dark cavernous room.

Inside, were a couple of young men. The space was dark enough that I pulled my flashlight from the hip holster and held it up into the ceiling for some way to illuminate the faces and the space. I immediately felt uncomfortable, as I was not sure who these men were and why were we brought to this place.

"These are the bean police," Felton explained as he introduced the two men who looked like thugs from a local gang. "Their job is to watch these women count every pail of beans that we will put into the bags so that we are not shorted. I will be watching for any bad or rotten beans, as some of the vendors here are known for topping of large bags of rotten beans with a few inches of good beans and selling them at full price."

The two hundred pound bags of beans were dumped onto a large tarp on the floor while new plastic coated large bags were brought out to load. With each ten pails of beans that were deposited into the bag, Felton would pick up a bean and put it into his hand to keep count. It was primitive, but then again, we were in a primitive market and it was working and quite intriguing.

When the counting was complete, large needles made of cow bone were brought out to sew the bags shut with plastic coated string. Money was to be exchanged; hands met to acknowledge the purchase and each man picked up a bag on his shoulder and carried them out of the room back into the sunshine.

Felton went to get the car with me trailing behind again, not to be left with the bean police who stayed behind guarding the large heavy bags that had just been loaded with this month's allotment of the precious food that would feed our children.

We returned within a few minutes and the young men loaded the bags into the back of the car, each being paid the equivalent of twenty cents for their work. Before we left, one of the women took me aside and asked if I could bring her something the next time I was at the market.

"I need vitamins please. I can't afford them," she explained.

We had many bottles of adult vitamins in our bags, and I thought we could spare at least one bottle to give her. I didn't ask why she wanted them, but could see by looking into her eyes surrounded by the dark circles and her thin body that she was serious about the need.

We got into the car surrounded by the vendors who had taken notice of the white woman spending time with the woman who sold beans. The fact that I took the time and embraced her as I left sent a visual message down the open market of the city. It was intriguing to them, and was what I needed to do.

"She has HIV/AIDS and is taking ARVS," explained Felton, as we left with the beans. "It would help her a great deal if you could provide that medicine for her."

I was more than happy to give her the vitamins. I watched her wave and watch us as we drove away. Life here is tough.

From there we drove to a station that sold gas, soap, cooking oil, and eggs. This time we purchased soap and cooking oil and left with a small hand written receipt. No soap or cooking oil police were required. We headed out of town and back to the OMNI school, ready to provide this week's food for the children. The car was overflowing with food that would fill the little bellies of those who were so desperately hungry and waiting.

Years of hard work, dedication, and sacrifice continued from this point on. I have to admit that when my family, or my friends or even the public thought I should quit and leave Africa, I listened, felt pressured, but did not give up on my calling to serve in Africa. Many sleepless nights over fifteen years arrived at the most inopportune times. When I thought that I could not do this any longer, often times alone, God provided another ray of hope, another donation, and another person who stepped forward to support our cause for the children. The land that was donated eventually became our home. It is the small sixty-acres that OMNI will do whatever we can to provide for the children who have no future without this site to educate them, feed them, clothe them, and heal wounds and illnesses as they arise. Our staff has been an evolution of local people looking for work, looking for purpose and finally realizing that we care for them. It is not a job, but a family.

Be Lovely

Jim was now beginning to understand the nature and characteristics of our travels and of the African way of doing business. In this part of the world, time has little value. The focus is on the event and not necessarily when it happens, but if it happens and who is present.

We were flying over once again to check on the new school building project. Upon arrival, Felton mentioned that despite the building progress, the villagers of George, just down the road from our site, were becoming impatient with what to them appeared like a lack of "rapid progress." I wondered why a group of villagers could feel this way when nothing had happened in this village to make a change in centuries. Our project was the first of its kind, and progress was indeed being made. Children for the first time were attending school and getting an education. Those same children were receiving a full hot meal every day, wearing a uniform donated by OMNI and receiving medical care when needed. Apparently there were expectations, real or not, that had failed to be met.

Jim still traveled with an abundance of clothes, which, to my amazement, were pressed and stylish. He had plenty of electronic gadgets and computers to keep him occupied and organized. His flashy wristwatch made him a target for theft. Not wearing expensive items was one of the many points that I had made in our team training. Obviously he did not listen. He also carried a 35 mm camera, complete with a long lens, for recording the events of the day. All of this was compiled in his backpack which he carried with him every day with great ease.

Felton drove up to our site where we had been reviewing the building plans to announce that the villagers in the compound were gaining in number and were becoming increasingly angry. They were demanding that the president of OMNI come and speak to them about the lack of progress in their village.

He then drove the Land Rover to Jim and I at the meeting site - the village center. The center was composed of a twelve-foot high cement block wall surrounded by a cement building painted in a beautiful ocean teal that was now peeling. An enchanting courtyard with a few mature trees, two out houses, needing emptied, and random plants scattered here and there. Unfortunately, the water in the well was contaminated, but all of the villagers, about 400 in all, brought their vessels and containers there for water. Some people brought their tin bowls that carried the beans from the fields for washing.

As we entered the metal gate, that had been unlocked by one of the village leaders, we drove into the enclosed courtyard. Organized in a very large circle, two and three people deep, were about 250 villagers. In the center of the circle sat a small wooden bench about four-feet long. Felton motioned for me to enter the circle and have a seat so that I could address the angry crowd. I turned to Jim and said, "Let's go in and get this talk done."

Jim took a good look around at the restless and agitated crowd and came to his own conclusion of how this should be handled. "I think that you should do this one solo, Karen. I'll be happy to stay outside of the circle and take pictures."

How generous! I thought. His statement reminded me of the Roman Colosseum where they threw the poor souls into the lion's path for consumption. With that, he and his camera were gone and he removed himself clearly from this scenario.

I didn't have much of a plan at that point and again had visions of a new soup recipe that had consisted of stone soup, soon to be revised by adding 120-pounds of white meat, a few onions, and tomatoes, and there was dinner. People would miss me at home, I hoped, but the good news was that Jim would have it all on film for their review.

With no time left and no escape plan, I decided to hit this head on as I usually did with challenges. There is no sense trying to avoid it. I would just have to address this crowd and do the very best that I could to explain our good intentions. I turned to Felton, who was going to be my interpreter for my speech and asked, "Please, Felton, what advice do you have for me in this situation?"

Felton was Zambian, intelligent, and had a pretty level head on him. I expected that we would sit for several minutes and go over the game plan, perhaps even review key names and leaders within the village that I should address. We would go over tribal protocol and any other beneficial acts of graciousness that I could bring forward. Felton would direct me in his plan that would explain all of our long range goals, and projects, and keep me safe. I anticipated his directions.

"Be lovely," was all he said.

"That's it!?" I asked. "Are you sure?"

He nodded and motioned for me to go into the human circle - a complete 360 degrees of angry African people. The view looked the same no matter which way I turned. Angry faces focused on me, the hub of the circle. If they wanted to attack, I was in the perfect spot.

I began my talk, thanking everyone for coming, being sure to pause to allow Foster to interpret my English into tribal Bemba. *I didn't invite these people, and I sure didn't want to be there*, I thought with great panic as my heart pounded in my chest.

'Be lovely,' echoed in my ear. 'Be lovely,' he had advised.

"I am so happy to be here with you and appreciate all of your time and attention. It is with great honor that

I come before you and tell you how much this community and your children mean to us. We remain dedicated to this region, the people and your well-being." I stated as I watched the crowd surround me like a circle of death.

We think of you each day and plan to be here for a long time, enhancing your village and moving forward with education and medical care." I saw few smiles even with this statement.

My talk continued in the same manner for over twenty minutes until I could see some smiles in the crowd.

As I concluded my talk, the women starting trilling with their tongues which was a sign of approval. The men clapped and nodded their heads. It was at that point I suspected that the menu for the evening had reverted back to vegetable soup. There would be no meat this time.

I curtsied and walked out of the circle, where Jim was waiting with his camera, long lens extended as he had taken pictures from a distance, and had recorded this entire unbelievable, threatening experience. "Karen, you didn't say anything. Your message had no content." Jim correctively commented as he showed a visible face of disappointment.

"I know," I said with a smile. "But I was lovely, and that's all that we needed."

We got in the burgundy car with our driver and drove away.

Jim was now gaining confidence in traveling with OMNI to Africa and his position on the team now included board member. Within a year, he was nominated and voted to be vice president. His responsibilities for travel increased and his fear of the unknown seemed to dwindle.

We were invited to Nairobi, Kenya on our way to Zambia, the following year by Father Gary a priest who had dedicated his life to working with the poor. As most who are authentic in their faith and their service, he was loved by his parishioners and by the villagers where he lived.

Father Gary lived in a large rectory along with about fifteen other men of the cloth who worked endlessly for the underserved and indigent population. Upon arrival in Nairobi, we were picked up by a driver at the airport and made the hour long journey after sunset through the city, explosive with cars, over packed buses, and loud noises coming from blaring radios. Again, we had no idea where our actual destination would be, but felt safe knowing we were with this young priest.

We arrived late at night to a large building surrounded by electric gates and barbed wire. As our car entered the security barrier, we saw lovely grounds wrapping a stark building where the priests live. We were escorted into the building and taken up to the second floor where light, laughter, and the sound of a television escaped from the thin wooden door.

We found the living area of the austere structure where all sense of formality was left at the door. "Come in and welcome to our home," announced one of the priests sitting in an easy chair watching the news, beer in hand. It was a small room, gray and pale blue in color, with a few sofa chairs and a couch set haphazardly around the room. Just to the left as we entered was a small metal table with beer, wine, and come mismatched glasses.

"You must be tired from your long flight. Would you like a beer or wine?" another asked. We spent about an hour with the priests hearing story after story of their encounters with the poor within Kenya and the difficulties and dangers that came with it.

Just prior to our arrival that week, a nun, from the same order, had been brutally murdered in her home. The motive was unknown, as theft was one of the details of her gruesome demise. Security had been heightened at both of the homes and tensions were running high as no individual or group had been arrested in this horrific tragedy.

Stories unfolded of the poor coming to the gates of the rectory asking for food, clothing, and assistance. Each time, their wounds were tended to, bellies filled, and shoes and clothing provided. Lives were cared for without even leaving the confinement of the building.

The prayers of the evening proceeded the dinner of chicken, greens, and potatoes. We were each escorted to our individual rooms down long barren halls that had no decorations or character. I was shown to my room of 1H, second to the last door on the right before the hall turned left to the large bathroom and showers. Being the only woman in the building I had the whole wing and bathroom to myself. I could hear my footsteps echo and bounce off the barren walls as I clutched my flashlight, and travel bag to head to the showers.

My room held a single bed with a metal frame, one small wooden table, a bible, and a sink. I wondered how it would be to live here and feel that sense of extreme isolation. Maybe some liked it, but for me, it felt lonely and extremely barren of the warmth that the community of friends and family would have.

The next morning a simple breakfast or coffee, water, toast, and eggs was served and we were off in Father Gary's SUV bound for Kabera, the largest slum dwelling in Africa and the second largest slum in the world. The population is a vast million plus people occupying just a 6 percent of the land in Nairobi. The Kenya government owned the land.

As we made our way up the dirt road, littered with garbage and paper, and piles that smoldered in the hazy sun, we found a small place to park the vehicle. Father Gary's instructed us to leave all bags, cameras or any valuables in the car where the accompanying priest would stay and guard it for us. As we came to the crest of the hill prior to our descent on the goat path into Kabera, we stopped to look at the horizon of tiny mud shacks, with tin roofs built so tightly together that you could not see the ground between. The shacks were as far as our eyes could see from the left to the right, dense
dirty and defiant of any comfort. It looked like an open sore on the face of the earth, populated by humanity with little hope of ever healing.

The path going down was packed dirt and rock, and we descended between two limestone walls that could be touched easily if you extended your arms. They looked like goat paths, but no goats were seen as they had all been consumed in this dense populous of extreme poverty. There is no electricity, no plumbing, and no clean water.

"Be careful where you step," said Father Gary. "You might step on some of the flying toilets here." The flying toilets were tiny worn plastic bags of human waste that after being used were tossed wherever they landed, which was just about everywhere. The stench was gagging.

Each hut was no more than 10x10 with a small hole absent from the mud walls, which served as a window. The tin roofs were worn, mismatched, and patched with stones and plastic. As many as eight to ten family members slept, ate, and lived in these deplorable conditions. There is no education for the children and no recreation. Glue sniffing and various other street drugs become a way to numb themselves from the gravity of their situation. Hope is nonexistent.

Gangs in this settlement were common and we kept our eyes focused on Father Gary for instruction. Tension, especially at night between the Luo and the Kikuyu (the majority tribe), were high. Unemployment, except for small shop owners and some peddlers, was the norm. With lack of employment, comes alcoholism and outbursts of violence, rape, and other acts of crime that start early in the morning secondary to the consumption of Changaa, the local brew. Disease, illnesses, lack of sanitation, and health care is inconsolable even with attempts of assistance. Typhoid and cholera runs rampant among this population due to the contaminated water that runs from only two pipes to serve over one million people.

"We have tried to come here and help with the medical needs which are endless, but our nurses can only carry a few aspirins or bandages in their pockets - no large medical bags as they would be stolen," he explained. "We are hoping that OMNI will come here and provide a medical clinic that is desperately needed."

Jim and I looked at each other, knowing of the risks to the team would be extremely high and dangerous. We walked a little further and were asked to enter a home in Kabera. The entrance was a ragged cloth that hung from two mismatched nails, bent and rusted inside. It took a while for our eyes to adjust to the darkness. When we could finally see well, we found a young girl about nine years old caring for her little brother while their mother was out in the city trying to find food or work. There was nothing in the shack but a rusted tin coffee can that held a broken plastic cup. A burlap sack on the floor substituted as bedding for the family of three. Both children were sick and had no food. The father had left years ago. The temperature outside was rising, and so was the stench and the density of the air. I wondered how anyone could survive here and knew it would only be by the grace of God.

Father Gary handed a small amount of money to the young girl to give to the mother when she returned for food. Handing money over could only be done in the privacy of a home as the danger out in the open would be too great. We parted, saying our goodbyes, knowing that we would most likely never see them again. We made our way up the limestone goat path, through the flying toilet field and up to our waiting car.

Jim looked at me and said, "We are not going back there."

I agreed, as the danger for the team was too great. As president and team leader, my responsibility was to provide safety for the team in any of our missions. This was one time that safety was nonexistent and would be impossible to provide.

We made our way out through the mountains of burning trash piles, with heavy hearts and minds as we saw more children with swollen bellies and bare feet than we've seen in one place yet. We left a small donation with Father Gary that would support the wonderful work that he and his brothers in Christ were doing at the daycare center they ran, and for the shop where they were teaching carpentry skills accompanied by large doses of hope that gave dignity to these poor people. Our flight was later that afternoon, taking us on through Malawi and into Zambia once again.

Darkness Enters and Joins Darkness

Doreen had an uncanny way about her. With the sole intention of manipulating and massaging the truth much like layers of an onion peel, she knew when it was necessary to be charming. To get to the authentic version of the story, you would have to remove layer after layer of mistruths and deception. Honesty was in limited quantities and trust was fleeting. Stories of hers did not quite add up; she always managed to have some sort of explanation that covered the magnitude of her lies.

Red flags waved in my head each time she offered another layer of the onion of deceit.

Doreen had a dream or a scheme to have 1,100 children in an orphanage in Africa. Those were the exact number that she mentioned. She had no plan like the Swindle Brothers, however, the plan sounded like an amazing accomplishment if she could pull it off. When asking how this plan would come to light, there was no business sense, no concept of how one would feed, clothe, educate, and care for spiritually and medically. Her pipe dream was all smoke from what I could tell.

Her movements were questionable to say the least. She was in places that would enhance her well-being and livelihood, but did not sustain children in desperate need of the life sustaining necessities. She came into town and would stay with wealthy business people who took her in assuming her stories of woe and passion was true. Having strong sociopathic-like charisma, she managed to extract what she needed for herself and a few small things for the children.

After receiving the land from the chief of the region, her grandiose ideas grew, but with little planning or structure to back them up. There was never a doubt the children of this remote area needed food, health care, and education. Until we met her, Doreen used their needs to provide for her own selfish gains. The need grew for the children and so did the passion to create sustaining care for the extreme vulnerable in Africa.

When challenged about her plans to provide for the children, Doreen finally gather eighteen young boys, all needing a home, nutrition, and an education to her property to provide the care that she had talked about for so long. Some were double orphaned, and some remained with only one parent. There were children who had mothers who wanted relief from the daily obligation of feeding another mouth. This often happens in larger families suffering from extreme poverty, leaving more food for the rest. For the most part, the boys were healthy except for scabies and basic health care, lack of clothing, and education. All were extremely undernourished and lacked healthy development.

We agreed to support her efforts to provide for them with monthly financial support that came in the form of bags of meal, cooking oil, fish, flour, and sugar for breads, and clothing for each child. Working to support a mission from the other side of the world requires checks and balances. For every dollar we sent, we required receipts, and accountability. It seemed to work, at least in the beginning. For the first time, these children were getting three meals a day and a place to call home.

We shipped overseas containers holding 200,000 pounds of building supplies, medical, and educational supplies as well as clothing. At the bottom of the container were building supplies that, with our team on the ground, would erect two beautiful homes in ten days. "Out of Africa" and "Field of Dreams" was built on the Agape grounds. Within a few weeks they housed eight boys and two caregivers in each home, complete with bunk beds, dressers, clothing, and supplies for each child.

The chief came to personally dedicate the buildings and bless the work that OMNI had done. Dreams on all sides were coming true. The boys had a home for the first time.

Before our team could return, funds were wired to complete a new cafeteria made of cement block. A shower house was constructed that allowed children to come and bathe. There was no running water, but the structure allowed for privacy to bathe using a basin with hot water heated over the campfire.

I had the distinct privilege to bathe in this structure while serving on the medical team one year. A large basin of hot water was placed in the cement building that had two separate units, one for men and one for women. Each side was approximately six by eight feet, with a small open hole in the corner where the water could drain out into the yard.

There was no electricity, so upon entering the building at night, you could place your candle or flashlight in a corner. A small tin cup was given to dip into the water and pour over your body as you stood outside the basin. Once wet, one would lather up, and rinse with one or two more cups of water. The final cup was reserved to wash out your socks in water with whatever small amount of water that remained. Care was taken not to double dip into the basin as there were two more people who had to use this water before another basin would be brought in. I figured out that the second person was the coveted spot. The water was not boiling at this point and not cold as the third person experienced, but somewhere in a comfortable in-between. Wet hair and our laundry had to dry in the cold evening air. Once showered, we put on whatever clean clothes we had, dry socks, and our boots. We usually slept in them all to keep warm until the sun brought more heat in the morning.

The second year, we shipped another container from the U.S. that carried large blue metal building materials on it along with furniture, clothing, books, wheelchairs, and crutches for local hospitals and more. Hospitals in the U.S. had donated old metal cribs that were no longer in use. Babies would have a safe place to rest in the hospitals here that could not provide enough beds.

People on this side of the pond were excited to be able to contribute to the orphanage in Zambia and schools who needed community service were eager to offer students to help with packing and sorting. Groups of students earning public service hours and church members gathered on multiple weekends packing, sorting, and creating an inventory for the container manifest. Our last load filled the container to the very last inch, and was sealed with a handmade sign inside readying: "God Bless. Zambia or bust!" The doors were closed, sealed with a metal tie, and covered with a prayer for safe journey. Each container took us a minimum of three months to pack and several thousand dollars to ship to Africa.

Our medical team entered Zambia three months later hoping to coordinate our time there with the arrival of the container. The grueling flight that took two days with little sleep, flying through Nairobi, Malawi and finally into Zambia. We piled our gear and tired bodies into a rented bus, duffels in tow and headed north to the Mpongwe region with the destination of Agape Farm.

Our bags were packed with medical supplies, camping supplies for the team consisting of a bed roll each, and a camp pillow. There were no pillow cases as it seemed far too luxurious for this mission. My excuse was that it saved space and weight. Everyone's pillow was carefully marked with their initials on the "Do not remove tag, or you will go to jail." Once our heads hit the pillows at night, pillow cases were the last of our concerns.

Evenings at Agape in the deep bush was like being in a storybook about Africa. You could hear drums in the distance from small villages that gathered and sang around the fire at night. Smoke from the small fires rose into the sky trying to touch the millions of diamonds that God had sprinkled up in the heavens for us to see. The stars were brighter here and more beautiful without any unnatural lights dimming them. It is the deep bush, deep in the heart and soul of Mother Africa.

Eighteen small boys lived at Agape as their refuge getting fed, clothed, and receiving a Christian education in the school that we had built. OMNI provided funds each month for their food and education and whatever medical needs that they had. There seemed to be a sense of belonging for them, something that many of them in their short lives had not experienced. The older boys helped the younger boys and the staff watched over all of them.

We provided money for seeds to plant a garden and grow maize to help supplement the meals. The land was difficult to plow so we bought two donkeys that could pull a plow and dig deep troughs into the rich land. The kids named the donkeys Bobby and Tina and learned how to herd them into their huts built to contain them at night.

The next morning, while the oats cooked over the fire we heard a clatter in the distance. Seems someone forgot to latch the door on the donkey hut. Bobby and Tina took advantage of the mistake and ran through the grounds dodging the boys and kicking at anyone who got close. Bobby headed for the clothes line and with his big flat front teeth grabbed red shorts off the line, ran back into his house and ate them. The boys followed him, yelling, but it was too late. The shorts were history and the donkeys were happy with their great escape.

The following fall we returned with another medical team and arrived quite late in the deep bush at Agape. Something changed on the last trip in. Something had changed drastically, and it would affect the children, the land, and the mission. Evil had entered and met us in the dark of the night. We arrived at midnight after our two days of airline travel and an eight-hour bus drive. When I descended from the bus steps to greet Doreen, the only light came from the fire burning in the distance. I stepped into the presence of a man holding a rifle, with

Doreen standing next to him. "Well, you made it," she said in a cold voice.

I looked at the barrel of the gun just a few inches in front of me, at the man who held it, and then at Doreen. "This is an interesting way to greet an old friend," I responded to her.

"Well we have had some trouble here, and I have had some threats against me. I needed to protect myself," she said with an unconvincing tone. "We had a fire bomb thrown into the camp here and it burnt down my thatched roof over the cooking area. People are accusing me of things that I have not done." Her tone and body language appeared to conceal more than her words were telling us.

We were deep in the center of witchcraft country, but actions like this seemed to be more directed at her than that of evil pranks or the orphanage in general. My mind quickly formulated the problems that we were noticing over the last few months. Money had gone unaccounted for, things were costing more than before according to Doreen, and she was asking for more and more money than before.

It was late, and not much can be done with that late of an arrival. My immediate goal was to get the team settled into the hut, duffels unloaded and attempt getting as much sleep as possible before the rooster starts crowing at five in the morning. There was no need for an alarm clock here, and no need to worry about oversleeping.

The following morning, with the help of the rising sun, revealed our worst fears, far greater than money missing. The eighteen boys

arrived for their bowl of meal. Their clothes were soiled and worn beyond what they should be. Once smiling faces were void once again of happiness and bright eyes were now dull. In fact, their eyes looked downward and
they were fearful to come and sit near us as they usually did. Their symptoms were indicative of abuse. Once the meal was over, they were ordered by Doreen to march in single file to school. Our hearts sank as we watched the military line leave our presence.

Before we left that day for the clinic, a child ran to me and clung to my knees pleading to speak to me. He took the chance when Doreen was busy with another staff member on the property. Through our interpreter, the child spoke of lack of food, and substitution of boiled cabbage and tea. The meals that they had once known from OMNI were no longer being served. One child had been chained to a bed at night so that he would not run away. Others were forced to be Doreen's personal servants, emptying her bed pan at night and working long hours on the property.

With enough heard and more feared, we placed a complaint with the local police to protect the boys and arrest Doreen. The following day we had to fly back to the U.S. and could barely stand the thought of leaving the boys behind.

Weeks went by with no word from the officials or any action against Doreen until one day when I got a call from Felton. Doreen was called into the nearest town by an anonymous donor wanting to donate a truck full of supplies for the boys. She quickly went into town to receive the in-kind donations with intentions of selling them all on the streets for a profit. To her surprise, the police arrested her on the spot, and she was deported back to the U.S. within forty-eight hours. She had to leave Africa with nothing but the clothes on her back and the promise that she would never return to the country. We smiled and gave a sigh of relief for her swift departure. My next and immediate concern was the boys of Agape. Where were they and were they surviving?

The Agape Boys

Four boys ran as fast as they could through the dense bush in directions and destinations not knowing where they would end up. Their goal was not the arrival but the escape from the hands of abuse and cruelty of Doreen. Sometimes departures are necessary even when you don't know where you will end up merely to escape a dangerous situation.

Getting away was crucial in their mind and for their bodies to survival, even if it meant existing alone off the land. The boys who ran were skilled in catching small birds, what few there were, shooting them with homemade sling shots made from tree branches and pieces of abandoned rubber. Those who were not good shots used their skills with small rocks, killing mice and cooking them over an open fire created from small sticks and primitive fire lighting skills. Food of any kind was hard to find as the area was hunted hard by others who were equally as hungry. Those with some means dined on grasshoppers fried in oil. They had nothing. Oil, salt, shelter, and clean water... these were luxuries that they did not have. Once more, they would go without food or shelter. Having nothing once again was better than the abuse that they left behind at Agape. Doreen had taken away what little they had and all that we had given them.

Tarry and Peter were picked up by Social Services the same day as the deportation of Doreen and were evaluated and taken to a compound that bordered the Congo. It was vaguely known to be an intake shelter for children needing a temporary home and walking distance from the main gate. That invisible border divided a peaceful country from one known to foster violence and corruption. Cross it one way or the other, north or south, could mean life or one's death.

By the time that I arrived back in country, the boys, according to Social Service officers had been at the orphanage for a couple of weeks. Felton, Jim, Mary Sue, and I went to the office in Ndola to seek information about the missing boys. We were escorted into a room that was an office for one of the people in charge. Chairs were lined along the back of the room and we were ushered to sit for the meeting. The air was tense and there were no social conversations.

Once our business team was seated, the door that we had just entered into the room was filled with social welfare officers who entered and filed behind us. The door was closed and there was no room for an exit. The interrogation began, and we were questioned for over an hour about our intentions, our involvement with the boys and our knowledge of the boy's locations.

After a long discussion, in depth interrogation of our intentions, we were given permission to travel to the remote property that supposedly was an interim transitional home for vulnerable children who were homeless. This is the first that I had heard of any such home in my years here in this country. We left in our vehicle quite stunned and apprehensive of what we were going to find next.

Jim, Felton, Mary Sue, and I drove many miles north toward the Congo border. As we drove farther on the dirt road the land became more and more isolated. We eventually drove up to the large electric metal gates of the estate that seemed to be well over fifty-acres of land. The electronic barrier the separated us and the two boys and our vehicle was about one hundred yards from the border of the Congo, making it dangerously close to serious trouble. The road ended abruptly and brush and elephant grass lined the border. There was no visual crossing.

Behind the gates sat a guard hut manned with an armed guard. He exited at the same time as our car entered the property. We were motioned to drive in and park inside the gate just a few feet from its entrance. No sooner were we inside the property, the large metal gates began to close quickly behind us. The guard asked for our ID, of which we also offered our passports and business cards stating our purpose in this country. Our explanations that we were here to see our two boys seemed to fall on deaf ears.

This interesting interrogation to discover who we were and what our purpose was, fell on deafening silence across the property. There were no children to be seen or heard. In the distance about a quarter of a mile into the property and down a well-groomed road arose a large home, complete with a veranda and banana trees lining its front yard. I strained to hear voices of children but could not hear one. I kept looking to the right, just a few yards away and the dense trees of the Congo. Was this location a front for child trafficking into that dark country? Were the boys already gone, transported to another hell on earth that they could not escape from?

While my mind raced at the dangerous possibilities that these boys and now us were facing, a four-wheel drive vehicle came tearing down the road from the house, leaving a billowing cloud of rolling dust in its path. The guard had radioed the homeowner to come and further intimidate and interrogate us. His entrance was quite dramatic, aiming straight for us and stopping just a few feet from our vehicle where we stood as hostages inside his property.

"Who are you and why are you here?" He screamed at us. "I know people like you who come and steal children! Is that who you are and what you are up to?"

He was a white man, tall and about forty years old, with an obvious command of power among his staff and indeed the current situation that we found ourselves in. He demanded more identification and information of who sent us to his property. I noticed a large pistol with a wooden handle on his right back hip just under his jacket.

"We just came from the Child Welfare Office in Ndola," I began to explain as I felt I should take some control of what was going on if that was even possible. Having the card of the officer that we spoke to earlier in the morning from the welfare office, I pulled it from my pocket to show our authenticity.

"I don't believe you and only believe that you are here to steal from me," he growled.

"Felton, please get the welfare office on the phone and have someone verify our visit this morning and that we are here to see Tarry and Peter," I said.

Felton rang the office and got a receptionist just back from her lunch break. Our less than gracious host grabbed the phone and asked if she knew us. The answer was "No."

Of course it was going to be no! We didn't know her either! The end button was pushed on the phone and the line went dead. I expected that we were next and no one would ever find us. We were deep into the countryside and way too close to the Congo now for our own comfort or our own good.

Rapid conversation went on between Jim, me, Felton and our less than charming man who was determined to have us taken down in some way or another. I looked at Jim and thought, *Here we go again. I don't think any of your words or gifts will help on this one.*

Things got worse before they got better, and the conversation rapidly stopped as our big guy got into his vehicle. As quickly as the gates had closed behind us when we arrived, the gates started their clanky noise and opened up. The guard told us to leave. We had no problem getting into our vehicle and backing rapidly out of the tall gate.

"Drive fast Felton and don't stop until I tell you!" I cried.

He did.

We drove with no one saying a word until we were several miles away, yet still on a remote one lane dirt road. Felton stopped the car and fell back from the steering wheel and took a deep sigh.

"What was that all about?"

"We just barely made it out of there!" I announced.

Felton in his typical signature fashion, turned to me and in a very calm voice said, "God is not done with you yet." He put the car in drive and we drove off. I turned to Jim who was in the back seat, somewhat ashen yet from the experience that we just had. We just smiled and both said, "I think you are right."

It wasn't until we got all the way back into town that Felton pulled over and started to reveal his suspicions of the owner of the property. Rumors in town were circulating that they were Satan worshipers and had been involved in some child abduction and ritualistic activities. Their reputation was cloudy and like many stories in Zambia, could not be proven, but was placed in the evil category of life.

The character of the landowner certainly was not kind and loving, so we really had nothing to go on but our own experience with him. Another trip to the Social Welfare office was next on our agenda so that we could relay our strong concerns for the welfare and location of the two boys.

To our surprise and an answer to many prayers, the boys were released to our custody the following week. Their mother was provided a modest home near our school by OMNI, where rent and food was provided every month. Both boys attended our school every day and ate a hot meal at noon. Both grew taller than their original fate had allowed. Each time I would go to the campus, we made eye contact and I greeted them with a hug - which they returned, despite cultural norms. They had been rescued and given a chance at life of which we thank God for every day. Tarry graduated from the seventh grade at our school and Peter graduated two years after that. I often think of them as the Agape boys, and know that God is not done with them either.

God was done with Dorren's stay in Africa however. After many months of planning and investigation within Zambia, her rapid deportation back to America was swift and well-deserving. No one has heard from her since, and her damaged and tarnished reputation lingers deep into the bush. We left Agape Farm to the locals and the Chieftainess who ruled over that land.

Three years later, Dr. Henry and I made our way back to Agape Farm to see what remained. Overgrown bush grass claimed the dirt road and the fences collapsed. The huts that were so beautiful at one point in time were caving in from the heavy rains and lack of maintenance. The livestock was gone, the tractor had been removed, and there was no sign of life anywhere. The campfire that we used to sit around at night was cold and leveled to an ashen dust.

The orphanage that we built down the road was still standing, and we could see clothes drying on a bush near the building. A man and his wife, carrying a baby on her back, exited from the structure and carefully moved towards us. Within a few feet of us, smiles came across their faces and a hand was extended for us to shake. Webster was the last remaining staff, now hanging on to life by using the shelter that was once built for orphans. Our greeting was bittersweet. We left shortly after, having given our last gift of a small bag of rice that we had in the back of our vehicle. It wasn't much, but it was more than they had and could have hoped for that day.

With Grace

Years before the fall of Agape Farm, a woman arrived at our mobile clinic on an unpainted, handmade cart pulled by two large oxen. The large brown beasts with dangerously sharp horns came into our clinic site escorted by the owner who walked alongside encouraging them to reach their destination. At that moment, the oxen's purpose on this earth seemed to be elevated to the heroic task of delivering her to us without causing her further injury or pain.

The oxen cart represented the ambulance speeding down the highway in America with lights flashing and sirens blaring indicating that a critical patient needed attention and intervention in order to survive. The emergency here was represented by cumbersome animals, driven and directed by a switch made from a flexible tree limb, accompanied by a villager who was most likely their owner. Their heavy breathing, nostrils flared, and gate that pulled in unison was secondary to the massive weight that they shared. There was a hand carved wooden plank that served as a yoke that bound the two animals, creating a team. The wheels made an uneven sound of imperfect impact of wood meeting unpaved trail. The cart stopped and the oxen shifted side to side, forced to settle at this destination. The patient had been delivered. They were to wait in place until the switch would indicate another departure.

We had set up the clinic outside of the tribal hut at Agape. Our clinics, whether set in a building or an outdoor setting, always consists of the essential ingredients that will provide comprehensive care for most patients coming to seek assistance. Our intake position writes down the person's name, gender, and a brief complaint on a small history sheet similar to the size of a large postcard.

Once the person has entered our clinic line they are directed to triage, where either a nurse or a physician, or EMT will do another more in-depth medical and visual assessment of the patient and their family. Women come in with babies on their backs or wrapped in a small blanket concealed, and multiple children in tow.

Depending upon the complaint, the blood pressure is taken, physical, and medical history is documented, including last menstrual period, number of babies, is the baby moving if pregnant etc. From there the patient is directed to the appropriate physician such as an obstetrician, pediatrician, or internist.

I did a quick assessment of the back end of the cart, trying to see who was there, what was wrong, and if there was something that we needed to do immediately. I could see a small frail woman, lying on her back, propped up by a dirty blanket. She appeared to be about in her twenties. Her eyes were dark brown and teary. No sound came from her lips, but her face showed the lines one would have if you were in extreme pain.

From first glance, her upper body, head and arms had no signs of trauma. Her lower body, starting at about the waist, was concealed under a dome structure covered by a blanket. The physician and I pulled back the blanket carefully to reveal a birdcage type of homemade apparatus made of tree branches, stripped of their leaves. Its purpose was to keep the blanket and flies from making contact on her legs. Peering closer through the birdcage structure, we saw that her legs and lower body was covered by a lightweight cloth, saturated in body fluids.

The woman had fallen into a kerosene lantern while cooking and had suffered third degree burns from her groin to below her knees on both legs. Raw flesh and her knee cap were exposed on one of her legs. As medical professionals, your mind immediately moves into the mode of care and the plan of how to care for in the most effective manner. We were out in the bush, however, and all plans here would need to be modified in just about every step of the way. By all means, this woman should be in a burn unit and have a surgical team debride the wound in a sterile setting such as an operating room. We did not have those luxuries.

The mound of a small blanket, next to the woman's head, moved slightly, and the driver of the oxen pulled back the edges of the cloth to reveal a tiny baby. Our critical case load just doubled and our second patient was suffering from dehydration and starvation. She was four weeks old and had not eaten in the last four days since her mother's accident. Pain had separated them both from each other. Pain is invisible, yet the barrier kept a mother from even holding the child who desperately wanted her mother's touch and to be fed. Pain is the most unpleasant of our sensory abilities, and to keep herself protected from increased pain, she had to distance herself from her infant. Without our help they could both potentially die. I wasn't sure at that moment who could or would outlive the other, and for how long.

"Her burns are extensive, and I'm not sure what we can do here for her. She needs to be in a hospital and probably in intensive care looking at the extent of her burns," the doctor said. Joani was a trauma surgeon in the states, and had extensive experience in traumas of all types and origin. She came on the trip for the first time that year, thinking that she would be seeing cases of malaria, pneumonias, and such.

How much trauma do you see in the deep bush since there are no guns, no cars going down highways at a high speed? There are no motorcycle crashes.

This burn was trauma, and required care now, or she would die.

"What is her name?" I asked the driver through our interpreter.

"Grace," he replied.

"And the baby?"

"Blessing," he said.

God was grabbing at our hearts for sure.

"We have to do what we can with what we have," I responded. "What do you need to help her? And I will assist you."

Brian, one of our pre-med students on the team, put on a surgical gown and gloves and went out to the cart to bring our patient into the tiny clinic. He carefully lifted her from the bed of the oxen cart. Flies had already begun to swarm around the damp cloth that covered her extensive wound. The oxen driver, picked up the baby and watched as the mother was carried into the tiny clinic that was built just that past year. There were no lights inside, so it took a short time for our eyes to adjust to the less than optimal lighting inside. Rafters of untreated

154

wooden beams that had been hand cut were above our heads. There were wasp nests above us with the dull buzzing of the agitated creatures. I took note, and recalled that our epi-pen was somewhere out in duffle number fourteen. I prayed that I would not need to find it as I was allergic to their venom.

The cinder block building that was approximately the size of my kitchen at home was our clinic for the day should we need the privacy of a structure. The bulk of the patients were seen outside under the shade of the trees that surrounded the tiny building. We carried Grace into the building and placed her on the worn exam table that had been shipped from the U.S. on the last overseas container. There was no pull down roll of paper or a clean white pillow to place under her head. Blue paper operating drapes that normally would be used in surgery in the U.S. became the barrier between her and the clean but no sterile surface of the table. Cobwebs and spiders adorned the wooden beams over our head. Electricity was nonexistent, and we valued the sunlight that beamed through the tiny window near her left arm.

The list of items needed may not have matched what we had along in our duffels I feared, but we would do what we could. As a former OR nurse at the Mayo Clinic years before, it quickly reminded me of pulling packs and instruments in preparation for the surgical procedure. Only this time, we were pulling items from duffels that lay on the dirt floor and had no sterile operating room in which to lay out our supplies.

"I'll need surgical drapes, OR towels, a pair or two or straights, pick-ups, 4x4 gauze, a scalpel and handle, and plenty of saline solution," she commanded. "We need to gown and glove and prepare the table with drapes to lay the patient down."

Absent from the list, and most important was sedation. *Oh God, how could we do what we needed to do without providing her with any pain medication or sedation*, I thought.

We had no narcotics along, and no pain killers except Tylenol. I pulled the Tylenol from one of the duffels after finding it on the manifest, and gave her two 500 mg. tablets. Inadequate was the word that came to mind. One of the team members had kept a small wine bottle from the plane in his backpack and he quickly offered it up for this procedure. We opened the small plastic bottle of South African wine and let her swallow the pills. She winced as she had never had alcohol before. I so wished that we had more effective medication to give her. We didn't, however, and we did what we had to do with what little we had. It was a common and repetitive theme as you treat the masses from limited supplies.

The doctor had a small teddy bear that she had in her backpack that she had brought from the states to give to a child. It was apparently one that she had had for years and at one time meant something to her. She anticipated that there would be a child that was special to her, with needs that she felt were significant and would be someone that she could claim as her special child in Africa.

Joani had never married, nor had children of her own. She had worked, studied hard, and excelled as a medical student, and again in her residency. Against the odds, she would rise to the top in a predominantly male oriented profession. Dedication and commitment at this level of the medical profession comes with a price, and perhaps hers was that she would remain single and distanced from emotional relationships involving men. Maybe I was wrong, and perhaps there was more to the story that I didn't understand.

Our patient appeared to us like a child, small, frail, and in a life-threatening situation. Dr. Joani handed the small stuffed bear to the woman before she went to put on her surgical gown. No words were needed. The gift was like a universal language that spoke silent, unsaid words of comfort and empathy. She took the bear and hung on to it, keeping it close to her chest like a lost child left in the dark. She did not let go of it as long as we worked on her.

The procedure of debriding the wound, cleaning it and applying Silvadine, a medication that would assist with the wound healing, and applying clean dressings, took just short of three hours. Clearly what we had to do was painful and our patient deserved to scream and cry. Only a few tears slid down her cheek, and landed on the blue surgical drape under her thin dark brown face. Her eyes would stay tightly shut the entire time, except to open slightly to see if the little teddy bear was really still there. I imagined that even at the age of this young woman clearly in her twenties, the bear was her first gift, and she wasn't going to let go of it.

Brian had his first experience as a second assistant in this case and did very well. Joani worked methodically on one leg, starting at the groin, and working to the knee, then on the other leg in the same manner. One of the gifts that Joani possessed, I learned over the years working with her, was the calming force that she instilled in traumatic situations. It was as though the room slowed down to a pace that created a sense of control and defined precision. We worked as a team, with limited supplies, doing the very best for this woman that we could. There was no conversation except for requests for more gauze or saline.

I was grateful for Grace's sake when the procedure was over. Grateful that she survived it and apologetic in my heart for not being able to provide more pain control. Brian carried her back to the cart where we had placed a clean blue drape where her body was to lay for the ride to her hut, miles from our clinic. Detailed instructions were given to the man directing the oxen to return to us tomorrow at another location about 30 minutes from us where we would have to change her dressings again and clean more of the necrotic tissue damaged by the fire. We gave her a bottle of Tylenol and more bandages to reinforce any drainage that would occur during the night. All instructions were interpreted from English to Bemba through Phyllis the nurse of this tiny village.

We gave her dry baby formula and a bottle for the baby to the man at the helm of the oxen cart. Through an interpreter we provided him with instructions on how to boil the water from the stream first, let it cool, and how to measure the powder. He seemed to understand and showed gestures that he was grateful. The small can of formula had to save a life, and I prayed that it would do all of that. Without it, there was no chance of survival. We would hydrate the baby with an eye dropper filled with sugar and salt water, then eventually begin a feeding program with the formula that we had. Grace saw the handover, and her eyes lit with hope that her baby had a chance.

The cries from a hungry baby are never forgotten. To see a child too weak to cry from starvation is haunting. It stays with you forever. Grace's baby was there...too weak but still alive.

As the oxen cart was about to pull away, both of Grace's arms rose up from under the blanket and motioned for me. Once alongside the cart, I leaned over the wooden wall so she could whisper something to me.

"Thank you," she said in broken English.

Tears welled up in my eyes as I heard her speak for the first time that day. Imagine her thanking us for putting her through all of this. Astonished that she could speak English, I wondered if there was anything else that she needed. The driver motioned to the interpreter to tell us that she could understand some of what we were saying, but could not speak much beyond what she had just said.

"You are welcome dear Grace. You are welcome." The cart pulled away, and I know that a piece of my heart went along with her.

We treated her wounds three more times while we were in the bush area before we headed back to the compounds in the city. Each time the man led the oxen to our clinic site, pulling the precious cargo. Each time we went through the painful and lengthy process of debriding her hellacious wounds, applying Silvadine ointment and new bandages, wrapped with loving care. Each time, she offered thanks and a hug before she departed.

I carried Grace's image with me for years. I prayed that I would see her again, that she would survive, and that her baby would have enough food. The likelihood of each of those prayers coming true was slim.

Annie, Orphan of the Continent

In Luke 9:48, Jesus says, "Anyone who takes care of a little child is caring for me. And whoever cares for me is caring for God who sent me. Your care for others is the measure of your greatness."

My interpreter for the day was a young woman, thin and well dressed for the distant region we were in. She and the baby, that lay in her arms quietly all day, were noticeable for this village. I learned about Kasongo from one of my staff and it was described like this: "This is a village that needs help. There is no law and order as everyone gets drunk by nine hours. There is a small government clinic in the village that has been abandoned. The government is afraid to go back there due to the high level of witchcraft."

It was to be the immediate location on my radar screen and on my list for the next village for our team to provide care. Needs were great, no one would go there, and there was an element of danger that if harnessed, we could make it work. The most important note to register, was that there was need being unmet. We had to go there.

Our bus traveled west on a small tar road, turning left at the tree with three over-sized branches. This was a common mode of direction that I was not yet used to. From there, we traveled down an elephant grass-lined dirt road. A few people could be seen traveling on foot down this road to the main road in hopes of catching a ride to the nearest town which was thirty-miles away. Life here is remote, distant from all others and taken off the list of financial and hands-on support by the government. Left to disintegrate due to local brew that encompassed young lives, violated their families and ate away at their souls and liver, if they knew that they had one.

A once tiny three room cement building built perhaps by a grant from another country and endorsed by the government was deemed too remote, and too risky to continue support or care. They were left to their own demise. Imploding in alcoholism and witchcraft, poverty and lack of health care at any level - a village of unrest, violence, and despair. We would go there.

The mustard yellow chipped painted building, that was once a medical clinic, was standing alone in the run down village. The town ran rampant with children, goats, drunk young men and women tending to their babies at a very early age. Main Street was just a goat path and there were no cross roads that I could see except a few footpaths that meandered back to more poverty and misery.

We were an anomaly in this location. So out of context, so out of culture, and so out of the imbalance of life that hung by a thread for so many. Things here did not function well. Order was not the norm. Chaos and disorder was what everyone expected and knew.

My interpreter's baby lay wrapped in a blanket, held tight to her lap. This alone was a significant clue that this baby was not her baby. African woman would always carry and care for their babies by carrying them on their back and nursing them frequently. I took notice and although I was appreciative of her interpretation, kept my eyes on this beautiful baby. The baby was like a pearl, precious, single in its shell, and beyond measure was to be noticed and protected.

"Can I be tested?" the woman asked at the end of the day.

I knew what she wanted - to be tested for HIV was a common request for young people who were sexually active in a country where this disease consumed and took ownership of lives and futures. It was as though they knew that they would contract the disease, and getting tested was a perk in knowing when. It was a given, you would die from either malaria or HIV. Life had no boundaries as far as restrictions as everyone would die young. They were correct - life expectancy was only thirty-two. No one escaped this village without the exit card of death. There were no exceptions. There was no hope, the most significant element lacking in any society. We had to bring hope here.

The test trip showed positive, indicating a strong likelihood of HIV positive disease. Our physician delivered the news in a setting away from the crowds and preserving confidentiality. "There is a very strong indication that you have HIV AIDS, according to our blood test. We encourage you to seek treatment."

She was encouraged to go to the HIV clinic in town, to start on antiretroviral treatment, offered at no cost by the government. Further counseling was given on prevention of exposure to others, safe sex, and all that goes with diagnoses such as this. Henry, our physician and long-time friend prayed with her before she left, and our hearts sank knowing that this very young woman would be up against a life endangering disease here in Africa.

Her reaction was less than what I thought it would be. "Thank you," she replied softly. She walked away to absorb her news.

Before she left, I asked to hold the baby - Annie was her name. She was awake now and I had hoped that this slight offer to hold her would be a welcome break for this woman. Annie was handed over to me, and I cradled her in my arms, thinking about this beautiful baby, who had already lost her mother, and was in jeopardy of losing the only mother now that she had.

After a few minutes of being held and cuddled, Annie started to cry, not out of lack of attention, but a strong cry of hunger. I turned to her caregiver and said, "She is hungry and needs to be fed. If you give me her bottle, I will be happy to feed her for you."

From a small bag tucked under her wrap came a bottle filled with dark clear liquid. "What is this?" I asked, not recognizing this as any formula I had ever seen.

"It's black tea. And it's all that we have to feed her," came the reply.

I sent our driver into town with the funds and instructions to purchase canned, powdered baby formula and bring it back to us as soon as possible. Before we left the village, Annie was drinking white nutritious formula in the same bottle that once held the black liquid. Without calories and nutrients, starvation would have eventually taken her life.

Annie was our new baby, adopted in all of our hearts, yet a resident of this unruly village. Her life had become our responsibility, a mission that we took on with great seriousness and delight.

Our staff delivered formula at the first of every month to Annie's caretaker until I returned three months later on a business trip. I found Annie, but with great sorrow, we learned of another loss in her very young life. Her caregiver had died just a few weeks earlier, another young woman, gone. It illuminated a startling statistic of how HIV ravages the continent.

Annie had been placed with her mother's cousin and her husband. Pristell and her blind husband Frank had been asked to take on the responsibility of being parents to this tiny baby, a burden that they both expressed as perhaps punishment from God. Since Frank was blind and unable to work, Pristell would walk miles into the countryside and work as a day worker in a farmer's field, toiling long days at the end of a wooden handmade hoe. Having a small baby created a situation for them that was near impossible as they barely had enough money to feed themselves.

Realizing this difficult situation and wanting Annie to thrive in her new home, OMNI began delivering cooking oil, meal, candles, and kapenta, the small fish of the area, to them along with the formula, clothing, and blankets for Annie. It seemed to be working well, and Pristell, who had been unable to have children of her own, began to love Annie as though she was born from her. A family was created and there was love for Annie who no longer could fit the label of double orphan.

OMNI delivered food, clothing, cooking oil, candles and shoes, to Annie over the course of seven years. The dark interior of their humble and primitive hut was lit with the sound of this little girl who continued to thrive despite multiple cases of malaria every year. OMNI paid for her treatment, her vitamins, and the transportation money that it took to get her to the hospital miles away from her village.

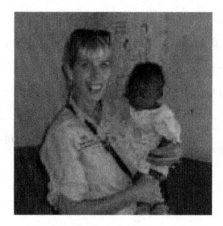

Anne of Kasongo

Annie was our magnet draw point each time our team worked in the village of Kasongo. We wanted to see the beautiful little face with the dark bright eyes from the good nutrition that we had been providing to her and her family. She recognized us from year to year, and eventually would walk up to us, standing near us, yet offering very little in words or emotion. Her adopted mother thanked us for her care, her food, and her clothing.

She hid behind Pristell's skirt when we would come to see her and she'd peek out from the safety of her surrogate mother just long enough to see that we were still there. From time to time, she would greet us in her native language and as the years went on, her words also included small phrases in English.

The poverty level in Annie's village is staggering, and people there survived on subsistence farming or working in the fields for

166

another landowner. Pristell often took Annie on her back when she was a baby and walked many kilometers to a field where she used her handmade hoe to till the dirt from sun up to sun down, walking home to sleep long enough to get up and repeat the labor the next day. It was just enough to earn some ground meal for her family to eat.

When we delivered food, we brought the small bags of meal, salt, and oil in through the back road so that the neighbors could not see the gifts that were arriving. Pristin often commented that she feared being robbed or worse simply because they had more food than their neighbors. Witchcraft loomed in the village like a dense fog hanging in a valley. You could sense it, but could not touch it or identify it.

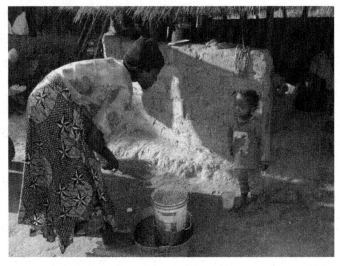

Frank was good to Annie, but Annie was clearly attached to Pristell and viewed her as her natural mother. Frank, although seeing impaired, wearing thick cracked glasses that resembled glass bottle bottoms, was quite cunning and crafty in his ability to work the crowd and make sure that he was personally well taken care of.

He often times would befriend members of our medical team during the clinics so that he could add or obtain items for his resources or for resale. He loved pens, small bottles of vitamins, bandages, sunglasses, and knit hats. These were items that could later be easily sold with little detection. Frank was outwardly smooth and had the ability to insert himself in situations where he would benefit the most.

Each year Frank showed up to volunteer at our clinic in Kasongo working as an interpreter in the pharmacy. He had the annoying presence to continually ask for items from our pharmacy table stating that his family, neighbors, or friends were in need of these items. On several occasions, my nurses would complain at the end of the day that he had helped himself via a five finger discount to various medications and items that were designated for the people who had no resources. When he thought that no one was looking he would pocket such items.

Frank was a petty thief, and possessed characteristics of deception. It was a constant struggle having him around and his presence was bothersome to us as we worked the long days serving the needs of over 600 patients a day. Items would go missing, and Frank's pockets were fuller at the end of the day than they were in the morning.

On one of our clinics, that took place in a maize field just to the base of the Congo hills and border, was finishing the day and packing up to head back to our accommodations about thirty minutes away. One of our team members was driving a vehicle and offered to give Frank a lift back into town and beyond into Kasongo. In the back of the truck were bags holding a dozen or more flashlights, batteries, and items to be donated later in the week. After Frank was dropped at his location, nearest the road to his hut, and our team member drove back to meet the team for dinner. The bags containing the flashlights were missing upon arrival to our lodge.

The following day, Frank once again volunteered at our clinic, our armed guards questioned him at the clinic about the missing flashlights, batteries, and other items, and not to our surprise all accusations were denied. Theft in Zambia is a criminal offense just as it would be in other countries, however, there, justice is swift.

A guard went to Frank's hut and found all of the missing items hidden in his small home. An arrest was imminent and indeed, within an hour, he was arrested and was taken to jail. We were hurt - shocked - as this was a man that had been gifted for years with food, clothing, financial support, and free health care for Annie and his wife, yet he chose to steal from us.

The same vehicle he stole from, drove him to jail. I was traveling to the clinic site in another truck and we met on the narrow dirt road.

The police officer had called my guard to alert us of the arrest and the intention to prosecute.

"Stop the car and please let me get out and address Frank before he goes to jail," I shouted as we narrowly passed.

The guard in Frank's vehicle got out and asked what we needed. I asked that they allow Frank to be brought out so that I could address him face to face before he was hauled to jail. A few minutes later, Frank stepped out of the back of the truck - cuffed and wearing a blue OMNI tee shirt, another gift from this mission.

I could hardly wait for him to come closer. "You have stolen from us despite our years of generous support, food, and care for your family. According to the laws here, you will be going to jail." My face heated with each word. "Officer, please remove his shirt, as the only OMNI shirt that will be in the jail is going to be on the team members who serve those inside. I will not have our shirt on a prisoner who has stolen from us!"

With that, the officer asked for the OMNI shirt to be removed. Frank took it off then he was loaded back into the vehicle. He spent two nights in jail and was released to his family, under the conditions that he would not be allowed to volunteer or steal from OMNI again.

We never saw Frank after that, but did hear about him years later. We were told that he later left his wife after beating her, fled to the capital. His profile as a thief remains as his legacy.

Word would come again and again that Annie had malaria. Another year would bring suffering as she was fighting off fevers, body aches, and enduring the treatment of the lifesaving medications. Her little body fought hard to survive. We continued to provide vitamins with iron as she became anemic several times, not wanting to eat or drink sufficiently.

One early morning, back in my office in the U.S., I opened an e-mail from Teddy, our headmaster, who kept track of the children that OMNI supported outside of our school compound.

"Dear Madam,

"I regret to inform you that our Annie of Kasongo has died this morning, after a brief illness and surgery.

Yours, sincerely, Teddy."

There was no other explanation, no details, just that Annie had died at the very young age of eight. My fingers raced across the keyboard to ask the many questions that were clouding my mind. *This could not be our Annie.*

"Are you sure it is OUR Annie of Kasongo?" I asked. "What did she die from, and with what ailment was she sick? Are you sure Teddy?"

A phone call from Africa later that morning confirmed the written words. Annie of Kasongo had fallen ill, two days earlier, complaining of severe stomach pains. She was rushed to the Children's Hospital and was evaluated. Her condition, according to the attending surgeon, was so severe that they felt she should undergo abdominal surgery to explore the etiology of the pain. The surgery was performed and she died the following morning.

OMNI paid for Annie's funeral and picked up her tiny body that housed her soul for eight short years. She was wrapped in clean sheets and a garland of fresh flowers encircled her little face before she was lowered into the ground. Pristell was devastated beyond comfort and once again, was childless.

Weeks later, while our team was setting up our clinic in the village of Kasongo, Pristell came to my station carrying the only picture that she had of Annie. Tears filled her eyes when she saw me and she wept quietly as I put my arm around her. This time, Annie was not hiding behind her skirt and she was there alone.

"There is something that you need to hear," Pristell whispered into my ear. "It is about how Annie died."

We moved away from the crowd and stood under one of the large trees. The villagers knew Pristell and could see that my concern for her was present.

"I think that Annie was poisoned by the witches," she said bluntly. "There were people who practice witchcraft that were jealous that Annie was ours and that she brought good fortune to Frank and me. We have been getting food and clothes for Annie and the witches are jealous." Her hands shook as tears slid down her hollow cheeks and onto the fabric of her shetenge. "There was nothing that the doctors could do once she had the poison in her."

Poisoning was something that we had heard of before and the witches seem to target children as they are the most vulnerable. It was devastating to hear, and unfortunately, a dark part of reality in this part of the world. Annie was gone and we could not bring her back. The Children's Hospital was the only medical facility for children in the region, and despite their attempts could not save this precious child.

The Children's Hospital is always full and for many is the last stop. My son Mark and I toured the five-story building years earlier to have a better understanding of the resource that was available to us as a medical team for admission of critical patients, too ill to be treated in the field by our team.

On appearance the hospital is bustling with people coming and going, walking in with children in various stages of illness. The emergency room is a small intake room with a tiny wooden table manned by a medical secretary. Backless wooden benches line the wall across from the inadequately-sized table and to the right were racks of handwritten files, overflowing from the frail metal frames. The admission process is laborious with every detail having to be written by hand, carbon copies creating a dim duplicate of the original paper.

Once that process has been completed, the patient and parents, are ushered through a small door where up to fifty or sixty patients sat along the walls on the wooden benches, unattended by any medical care. Children cried. Behind closed wooden doors on the left of us were the exam areas filled with cribs overflowing with children waiting to be admitted. During out visit, a mother could be heard wailing from the back room, holding her child that had just died while waiting to see the physician. Fresh paint had not covered these walls in years. Fear blanketed the air in anticipation of failed survival.

We had asked to see all the floors, being escorted by the director of nursing, who worked directly under the hospital CEO. Floor tiles were missing on some stairs, and the walls were in need of repair. Patient rooms were small housing up to four cribs, each with a child, some holding two due to lack of space. Windows in the rooms were cranked open to let in fresh air. Panes of glass were absent in several windows, and next to the void was glass that had cracked from years of use.

The orthopedic ward had no empty beds. Children of all ages lay on mattresses without sheets under them. The metal bed frames were chipped of paint and not all of the railings worked, exposing some small bodies to another fall from the bed. Mango trees were the main culprit this time of year, as children climbed higher within the branches to reach the

moist pulp of the fruit. Fractures of arms, legs and shoulders were common this time of year. Mangos were plentiful, and so were the injuries.

Adequate care to provide proper healing was painfully obvious. The femur is the longest bone in the body and, when broken, usually creates spasms of the surrounding muscles lending to a shortening of the leg and alignment of the bone would be impossible. Traction is normally applied to prevent the leg from contracting and shortening. Here the traction was created with a broken brick and rope that hung from the affected leg over the end of the bed. It wasn't the best, but it looked like it was working. It reminded me of my femur fracture years earlier and the difficulties I had even with some of the best orthopedic care.

Some of the children were fortunate enough to have received a cast - forcing them to bed for the swelling and pain to subside. I couldn't help but notice the little boy sitting in a broken wooden chair. The slats on the back held his swollen hand up. He was not as fortunate as he had been waiting two days to see the doctor with the hopes of getting a cast. We feared that he would need surgery as his arm was beginning to contract and the bone was clearly displaced.

On the floor at the end of the hallway lay a small boy, his mother next to him on a small mattress not large enough for either of them. His hand had swollen beyond recognition; the skin was tight from the edema. I asked about the little boy and what had happened to him and I was told that he was bit by a snake yesterday and was waiting to be seen by the doctor. It was a sight that no mother or nurse would want to see for any little child. We left money with the mother, just enough so that she could go outside to a street vendor and buy some food for both of them. Neither had eaten since the day before.

We made our way to the X-ray department. Benches full with waiting patients; staff occasionally entered and exited from the room. Above the door to the main X-ray room hung a sign that read: "DO NOT ENTER WHEN LIGHT IS ON." Detection of radiation useage was impossible as the light bulb had burned out months ago and was removed and never replaced due to lack of funds.

The pharmacy was a large room with freshly painted white shelves on three of the walls. The pharmacist, dressed in a white lab coat, shirt, and tie, stood proudly behind the open cutout where medications were dispensed. The shelves were almost bare except for a few bottles of Panadol (an equivalent to Tylenol), and three or four bottles of antibiotics. Handwritten labels, to identify medications, had been taped to the shelves usually slanting either to the left or right, but rarely straight. Above the labels were empty shelves capable of holding supplies, but today once again were empty.

We went from the pharmacy to the "SARA LEE High Cost Ward" where those families who had any money could receive care by paying cash. X-rays were $8.00 Surgical procedures were $42.00. Food was not available to the patients; family members brought it in small containers for the children. This ward was not as crowded as the others and the beds contained one child and not two.

From the high cost ward, down the stairs to the next level of the hospital sat the malnutrition ward. Children with advanced starvation, a common condition in this impoverished region, were taken for care. The

176

criteria for admission depended on the status of the child; each assessed by looking at the hands and feet, looking for swelling, which was actually protein breakdown from the body using the protein in attempts to survive the lack of nutrients.

Babies who are starving do not cry. They have no energy or strength to make any noise and lay motionless, with their large black eyes becoming the focal point of their emaciated face. Their silence is deafening. They lay on the beds weak and cheeks sunken from lack of food. The nurses on the malnutrition ward work extremely hard trying to save these babies. Each has a formula that they use to build back the nutrition in the child. Weights are taken every morning using a cloth sling hanging from a vertical scale. A watered-down version of porridge in small measured amounts are given to the child to start. Note is also taken to see how much the child urinates or wets the cloth beneath them indicating adequate hydration. Their temperature is closely monitored and their blood is checked for life threatening diseases that often times accompany the starvation.

Once the child can tolerate the watery porridge, the consistency is increased with more meal added to the solution. This may not happen for the first two weeks since the starvation is so advanced and their little systems have a hard time adjusting to the nutrition. All children are encouraged once they have enough strength to hold their own cup and drink what they can.

As we walked down the hall, a young mother sat on a wooden bench against the wall crying for the child that she had just lost. Through an open door next to her in the utility room where dirty pans, a mop, and a pail sat, was the body of her child, laid on the metal counter covered with a sheet. The mother was alone, and the child's body was alone, waiting for someone to make that final journey down the stairs to the morgue for labeling.

I didn't know this woman, but felt compelled to go and sit next to her, offering my sympathies and a shoulder to lean on. She cried, and slumped across my lap. We stayed with her for a few more moments until the nurse came to walk her and the child's body down the hall and out of the unit. Mothers holding their babies, just as close to death, watched silently as they observed what could very well be their experience next. Life and death existed in the same hallway. Absolute poverty was stealing another life far before its time.

The mortality rate here was high, and I asked to see the morgue, which was located in the basement of the hospital. It was noon, and as we descended down the narrow stairs and down a long dark hallway to the final door at the end. I imagined this descent to the basement being done with no elevators, and no gurneys to carry the deceased. Few people, except the man who carried the children's bodies descended to this level. It was the depths of the hospital and the depths of despair.

The nurse opened the large, heavy, metal door to reveal six shelves stacked from top to bottom with tiny bodies wrapped in white sheets, tied with string and labeled with the child's name, date, and time of death. The container was nearly full with the deaths from today and it was only noon. There were no sounds, no voices, only silence as we viewed the frail remains of these little lives. Today was their last day on this earth, and I prayed that they were now angels in God's care.

Bodies of these children that had been separated from their parents, waiting to be claimed later when some type of transportation could be arranged. For some, the body would be loaded on the back of a pickup truck accompanied by family members. For others, the tiny body would be draped over the back of a bicycle and begin its journey home for burial.

From there, they would make the agonizing journey to their funeral ceremony accompanied by wailing aunts and uncles, mothers, and grandmothers. For now, however, they were alone. Haunting. Rest in peace little angels. God is waiting for you.

These memories came flooding back as I envisioned our little Annie dying in the same hospital.

The details of Annie's death are still not clear, but rumor remains that Annie was poisoned by witchcraft, and succumbed to the evil that selfishly took her life. Jealousy is an ugly trait; retaliation in the form of death is evil.

Our little Annie was taken way too soon.

Before I Could Return: Haiti on the Fly

Back in the U.S. and working on all of the issues that arise daily in Africa is an ongoing task. The phone rang one afternoon and the agency from Colorado that cares for orphans and the poor in various parts of the world was heading to Haiti and wanted to know if I could accompany their team as they attempted to build a clinic in the distant regions beyond Port au Prince. I said that I could fly to Haiti and meet the team there. The time was short, in fact, it was the following weekend. I would be traveling alone this time.

I looked on the website for Haiti to see what the travel advisories were, and there was a posted alert for travelers: Beware of thefts, violence, and unrest especially in the city and the remote areas that lacked police presence. It was somewhat usual in Haiti for the most part. I knew that I was going in with an established team and felt like this was a viable trip and that, with my experience, I could contribute to the mission at hand. The team would meet me in Haiti, I just had to get down there and make the connection.

A team flew in from the western part of the U.S. and was going down to build a medical clinic and establish their mission. The other parts of the mission were to determine what else needed to be done in the immediate area and where the areas of most dire need were located.

My oldest son was in graduate school across the country a day's plane ride away, and he was the most likely person that could accompany me short of hiring a personal guard. He was well-traveled, up for adventure, and most importantly strong, street and travel savvy.

"Hi Scott, it's Mom. What are you doing next weekend?" I asked casually.

There was a brief pause before he answered as I could visualize him thinking of what was coming next. It was evident in his response that he knew me well, and asked, "Why? Where are you going and what are you up to now?"

I giggled. "I was wondering if you were free to go to Haiti with me. I need a bodyguard, and thought of you right away." I thought that this was a smooth entrance into this subject and perhaps he would agree. "I will meet you in Miami, and then we will fly down to Haiti together. I'll take care of your expenses, just need to know if you can and are willing to come along."

"Mom, I knew this was more than just a 'how you are doing call' and 'how is school'," he said. He seemed game to go but we had to talk about a few details. We talked awhile longer, more on logistics, and what was needed. We concluded the conversation, and agreed to meet in Miami on Friday and take it from there. I felt comfortable now going into this unknown, with him. Scott would be there and we could both handle this.

The trip down was uneventful, which is what is should be. When we arrived, things were different, and the events of the day were less than lacking intrigue. The airport was chaotic and the temperature was as heated as the political atmosphere. Our team from Colorado met us in the airport, introductions were made, and we boarded a beat up bus that was to take us to our accommodations some ninety minutes away. As we left the unkept road from the airport, we spotted the bloated body of a dead man lying in the middle of the road. The stench was recognizable to that of a decaying body.

"What happened? Was the question of the day from everyone on the bus. The driver casually reported that the victim had been caught stealing something in this area and was shot and killed by the local police. His body was left for those to see as a reminder that there was law and order on the island.

Note taken and filed.

The group searched for a location to organize and house their ministry all while looking for areas that needed the most help.

Our driver took us to the city dump where there was a significant population of extreme poor who made their home in the rubble of the garbage. It was like going to a small city within a mountain of refuse and debris. There were meandering paths that wound through the trash, and what appeared to be communities of people of who lived there.

"Watch your step, and be careful of the running contaminated water here. It is the juice from the garbage that is flowing down toward the street," the driver told us. The pungent odor, and the site was deplorable, yet people lived here because they had no other place to go.

We walked up the first mound of trash on the trail to a shell of a building that had no roof and no doors. People had staged out a small area that they called their own, no bigger than a single bed. Each spot had its own personality and characteristic reflected by what pieces of debris that the person had found to create some form of comfort.

We saw a woman sitting on the ground next to a man's body that was partially covered with a torn blanket. Her back was to the man, and she stared forward, barely noticing our small group. Our driver asked her about her wellness and that of her husband. We learned from her brief statement that he had died the day before, and that she was waiting until Thursday for the truck to come to take his body away. It was Monday; she had three more days to wait. Sitting next to a corpse for three days and nights seemed unbelievable. We asked if there was something that could be done, but were told that it was the way it was here in the dump.

As we stood there, one of our team members started a prayer for the dead man, and also asked for comfort and strength for the widow. It was a very somber moment in the trip and as soon as he finished the prayer, a young girl came running down the opposite path asking for our help.

"A baby has just been born in the next group of people," she said. "Come. Please make sure the baby and mother are all right."

I was the only nurse in the group. Without hesitation, I quickly went to the new mother. She was lying on the ground on an old mattress. The baby still had wet hair and was wrapped in a dirty towel, alert, and appearing to have good color.

"I'm a nurse," I explained. "May I see your baby and check to see if he is breathing all right and if he is doing well?" I asked. One of the women nearby placed the baby in my arms. I could see that he was breathing well, and appeared to be quite normal, except for being tinier than the average newborn. The mother was also doing well, and appeared to be very young. Her boyfriend stood by her side and both looked as though they had little experience in taking care of a newborn baby. The new mother was going to nurse the baby, and after staying with them for about an hour, felt that both were stable enough to leave them and move to another site.

The agency that we were traveling with said that they would send someone out the following day to check on both of them and bring food and more blankets for the new family. Life in the dump was going to be rough and another generation was continuing on in the same squalor. They had found the site that would be soon under their care. The work here would be endless and plans to relocate the refugees there was soon underway. Haiti had new angels on the ground and the country would be better for it. More angels would be needed, and I prayed that they would come in droves to this land.

The night before we left, our team moved to an abandoned hotel site on the shore of Haiti. The hotel had at one time been quite nice, but was now more run down and seemed quite desolate in location. We did not sleep well that night fearing for the possible invasion of shore bandits. Theft coupled with violence was common there and this seemed to be a perfect set-up for this. Scott slept with his knife under his pillow. I was happy to know that he was not far away from where I was staying, and looked forward to our flight home.

Before we left the next day, we stopped at a small intake center for children who had been abandoned or displaced. That morning a small girl, around eleven or twelve, had been thrown out of the back of a moving pickup truck onto the highway in front of the center. Both of her legs were broken and she had cigarette burns on her body. This poor child had been the tragic victim of sexual and physical abuse for several months, and then discarded like a piece of trash before the center. We knew that she would be well taken care of here, but also were very aware that her emotional scars would never heal. We kept her in our prayers for many weeks after that encounter.

Within months of traveling to Haiti, I was back with a full medical team in Zambia and determined to visit each village that we had treated the year before. The rainy season had just ended and some of the roads were impassable and plans for a bush clinic were not possible. Rick had spent the day with the building team and had heard of a remote village that had never received medical care. "It's a surprise," he said. His sparkly eyes had more news to tell.

I don't like surprises.

The following day, we traveled to a village that had one main dirt road down the middle with small shanty houses on either side. It was typical in that it had no electricity, no running water, loads of kids running around the streets, goats, chickens, and a few drunken men. We had been given permission to set up our clinic in an abandoned church that had cement steps that lead up to a one room chapel. There were no benches but a few metal folding chairs and a table pushed to the side of the dark cement gray walls.

We organized the pharmacy table so that our backs were to the wall and used the only table available. There were a few wooden planks near the side of the building that had not been stolen yet and we propped them up on folding chairs to create a bench for people to sit while they were being examined. Our head lamps and flashlights came in handy when we poured medications and counted pills to fill the prescription.

Mark, my second son and his best friend Curt, were our crowd control that day, each standing six foot three and donning broad shoulders and seven-day-old beards. The crowds periodically became disruptive and violent at times as people pushed to get to the front of the line. I came out of the building to see how bad it really was when Mark took out the large pocket knife from his right boot and opened the blade. With a large stick in his left hand he began sharpening the stick with slow methodical swipes, peeling bark and wood chips as he progressed. He said nothing as his knife kept up the "crrrick, crrrick, crick" of the blade hitting the wood. The slower that he moved the blade, the quieter the crowd became. It worked like a charm.

At the end of the day, he had several sharp sticks, and we made it through the day with treating over 400 extremely needy patients. The villagers had been cared for and our team headed back into town for a much needed rest. Tomorrow Rick would reveal his surprise. I could hardly wait.

Our bus traveled west again paralleling the Congo border until we came to the Zambezi River where we turned south driving through the village that we had worked in the day before. We drove past the last house and into what looked like no-man's land as the road became a goat path that extended for another mile until we reached the end of the road and the banks of the Kafue River.

"So where is the village?" I asked Rick, looking at the rushing water in front of us.

"This is your surprise!" he exclaimed.

I looked around the banks for any sign of any houses. "We are going to portage across the river and set up a clinic at the island across from here. They have never had health care and it sounded like they needed us."

My heart leapt into my throat, and every part of me was saying no to this crazy idea.

The team started getting off the bus and looked excited at the prospect of taking a boat to the island. The problem is that there were no large boats around. The only boats were old wooden handmade floating disasters managed by the locals and would hold four to five team members and some gear per load. The wood that made up these floating oddities had never been painted and was worn by the African sun and water. To add to the joy, the boats all leaked, but were conveniently equipped with plastic gallon pails. These too had cracks in them and were used to scoop out the water at a faster rate than the water came in. Perfect. This was the last time that I would allow anyone to choose the site for our team.

The Kafue River is a major tributary to the Zambezi River and is the largest and longest river lying entirely within Zambia. Its water changes between slow flowing to fast swift channels and robust rapids. The river where we stood had a sandy bank and tall weeds covering most of the areas to our left and right. The river was known to be often occupied by hippos, crocodiles, otters and water monitors. Villagers had a healthy respect for the waters of this river as children and adults had gone missing secondary to crocodile strikes.

Felton turned to me and for the first time showed visible fear. "My people do not like the water, no water...no water."

"Well, Felton, we have to go across and you will be going with us," I said. "You will be all right and you can close your eyes if you want." As soon as I said that, it sounded ridiculous even to me, but it was the way it had to be.

We quickly chose small teams of three and four members to go across the river in each boat, selecting them according to weight and ability to assist in the event of an emergency. The boats did not seem as though they would carry any of us but we had to get the team over, now that we were committed to this clinic. We included in each boat two to three fifty pound duffels, carefully placing them in strategic places to balance the weight. There were also places farthest away from the water that was slowly leaking into the bottom of our vessel. Any excess supplies that were not needed were taken out to reduce the weight and the volume in the boat. We had to remind ourselves that wood floats and the journey needed to be as quick as possible to reach the other side.

I sat in a boat with one of the other RNs, one of the women who helped in the pharmacy. Our young man rowed as fast as he could and a smaller boy bailed water as it came up through the floorboards. It only took about three scoops before we were all bailing water to help stay afloat. The plastic pails were also cracked and leaked as we dumped water overboard.

The trip across took a few minutes, and we arrived on the shore of the small island. I'm not sure if that is good news or bad news, as we still had to cross back again at the end of the day, and had a full clinic to perform. The only benefit that I could see at that point is that we would have used up a great deal of weight from the medication and medical supply distribution, making our duffels lighter.

The team made it across and found the villagers of this small island to be more disruptive that we had the day before. The only flat, cleared space of packed dirt to set up the clinic was right next to the local pub which at ten in the morning was in full swing. A cheap boom box functioning on batteries was blaring into the African air and the home brew was flowing as fast as the river we just crossed. We could not hear ourselves think much less speak.

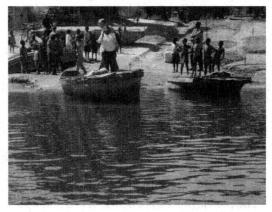

Old, wooden boat crossing the river to the island.

Rick made his way across the front of the small island to speak to the owner of the pub. He was good at public relations and negotiations, and this particular time we would need all of his skills. Within a few minutes, the music stopped and patrons staggered their way out of the bar and into our lines for medical care. Somehow, we often had inebriated clients in the clinic lines, and today was no exception.

"How did you get them to stop the music and clear the place?" I asked.

"It was easy," he replied. "I asked the owner how much a glass of brew was and how many did he think he would sell today. I did the math and bought out the bar for the day and shut it down." This transaction cost us $27.00 and was worth every cent.

The bar crowd mixed with the high population of practicing witches and organized witchcraft proved to make a challenging day for our team. There was little order except for the elderly women with walking sticks made from local trees. Wisdom and years of survival seemed to have infused a sense of calm in them. Each woman had lived through decades of devastating experiences and multiple losses.

Next to women with wisdom stood drunken mothers with babies, and men who were absent from their families. This proved to be our disorderly and inebriated group who lived in a constant stupor numbed by the local brew. No one stayed in lines and the crowd was loud and argumentative.

The oldest woman that we treated that day, however, was over 100 years old. She carried a government card indicating her citizenship and could not remember which month she was born or which year. She had a few teeth left and a smile that spread across her entire face. I wish I knew what her secret was as she appeared to be a happy soul. She had dodged the malaria and HIV bullet and survived longer than three generations after her. Her hands were gnarled and toughened by the

African sun, and her braided hair had a few tiny strands of silver. As the grandmother and matriarch of the family, she cared for five grandchildren, and was strong in her will and convictions to raise them. She was my favorite patient of the day and probably had more stories to tell than we had time to listen.

We packed up our duffels and made it to the shore of the island, ready for our return voyage back to civilization. The boats leaked and the plastic buckets looked worse than when we arrived that morning. The enormous African red sun was setting just over the banks of the river, and it was time to get off the water before the crocs came out.

Beyond the Savanna

Luke 9:6

They departed and went through the villages, bringing the good news and curing diseases everywhere.

Compelled to find her after two years, partly to see if what we did worked, but more importantly, to see if she even survived. I went back into the deep part of the bush, where small ruts and trails lead you deeper into witchcraft country. A place so far off the main road, hours in fact, where small African huts make up civilization as they know it. Wild animals are scarce here because they have been driven off or poached -

a place so remote that it's a miracle, along with a lot of prayers and "your time is not up yet" luck, to get you back out.

It is a location on the globe that has no concept of a crashing financial market, or the price of gold, or that Wall Street even exists. Currency runs in the form of goats, oxen, and skinny chickens. The wealthy have six goats, and perhaps a pair of oxen. Salt is a luxury and not many have it around. Goiters are common on the thin necks of the African women. Women and large bellied children have walked many kilometers to the small slow flowing creek to wash their clothes in the contaminated water under the African sky. They share the facilities with wild pigs that come to drink and bathe their dusty malformed bodies.

Life is simple, but not easy. The average life expectancy is now thirty-four, and those years reign heavy on their bodies, leaving a shell that appears far older than its years.

We stopped every few kilometers and asked villagers who were walking in the vast jungle if they knew of a woman named Grace who had suffered severe burns a few years ago. It's amazing to know that with a few descriptive adjectives and an explanation of why we were looking for her lead us deeper into the region where her home resided. My heart beat in fear of what we might see or not see once we arrived at her hut.

As we meandered further into the bush, the trail became less pronounced, and the trees coupled with termite mounds, became dense. We were to turn at the fork in the path, near the large tree, and go another kilometer. I saw smoke rising through the trees and knew that someone had to be alive there. It represented some form of hope for life. Someone was there and it probably was Grace. I would know her and with all reserve greet her properly with the Zambian handshake and bow, allowing her to respond if she wished with a hug.

We pulled up and saw that there were three small mud buildings, doors closed, and the cloth pulled across the narrow opening that functioned as a window. There were no people, and no sound of anyone around when we called her name. We peered into the window and saw faint shadows of bedding on the ground, and not much else.

A few feet away from the abandoned house was a small fire pit encircled with round, gray stones. Smoke ascended from the ashes, but there was no fire. Next to the stones laid a dog, left behind to fend for himself. His ribs were clearly visible, and his spine protruded from his emaciated back. He remained there and was unable to get up due to his weakened state. There was a cool pocket of air just before the fire pit that he was avoiding to keep warm. Smoke continued to rise. She had been there and had left just hours before. The homestead was desolate and bleak. There was no food anywhere - only a few piles of corn cobs barren of their fruit were left behind. In the corner sat a single shoe, worn beyond use and void of any laces. Its mate was nowhere to be seen.

I took out a pack of peanut butter crackers that I had brought from the States and opened it, throwing crackers to the ground where the dog laid dying. It would not save him, but I thought at least he would die having had the pleasure of eating one last meal. It was pitiful, and we were too late. Grace was gone and was probably in the same shape as the dog that was left behind. I could still smell the smoke as we got into our vehicle and looked back in the mirror to see it ascending into the sky.

The fire would soon be out.

And Especially Wife Number 4

None of us had the opportunity to meet her, and I doubt that we ever will. She has been prayed for everyday and remains in my mind like a ghost that haunts my thoughts and hangs there for more attention. I understand that she is a newlywed, young and naive of her place in life and her role as a wife. She probably came into her marriage accompanied by a dowry that her parents sent along with her. I don't know her value in amount of goats or cattle, but as wife number four, she was sought after by her husband as the youngest and the most desirable in the family. She came to the family, untouched, and pure. She now has HIV/AIDS and does not know it.

Polygamy in this part of the isolated country is common. So is the lack of education on how disease is spread. Families bound together by one common husband arrive with the same symptoms that have been spread to each other in their matrimonial beds. Husbands take in new wives, former sister in laws are married as a tribute to their late brother who also died of the disease. Multiple lives, infected by the same disease, producing the exact outcome marked finally by shallow graves and a handmade wooden marker. Children become orphans, who eventually share the same grounds, buried next to their mothers. The cycle continues and lives are cut short like mown grass.

I met wife #1, who appeared by all observations, to be the spokesperson for the wives. She came to us to be seen medically for peace of mind I suspect. She had been diagnosed in another clinic with HIV/AIDS and was on treatment as were her husband, wife #2, and #3. As she explained to me, they had made the decision not to tell the new wife of their diagnoses, keeping it their dark and dirty little secret. Wife #4 was never to know, and they would be the last ones to consider her in their agreement of deceit. The vision of the ostrich with its head in the sand came to mind. If we don't talk about it; don't look at it or deal with it, it won't be there. This is the ultimate mind set of being naive when dealing with this disease.

I spent a great deal of time with wife #1, encouraging her to discuss their diagnoses of this disease with wife #4, so that she could be tested and ultimately treated. I was passing judgment at this point, but I really felt, the poor girl had a right to know of her exposure and her fate, should she not be able to seek treatment like the three previous wives. It wasn't going to happen from the sounds of my conversation with wife #1. Honoring patient confidentiality, she left our clinic with her secret still intact. She had her vitamins, her Tylenol, and her secret all hidden from view of those around her. Until her disease becomes advanced, she will be able to conceal her diagnoses for quite some time.

The next morning our prayers started for wife #1, wife #2, wife #3, and especially wife #4. She will remain in our minds without a name, just "especially wife #4."

Under the Tree of Life, where wife #1, came to find refuge and medical help, came Skameezie, a seventeen-year-old girl who became paralyzed from the waist down when she was about seven when her sisters pushed the hand-propelled wheelchair that OMNI had provided for her several years ago. We moved her cart under the shade of the large tree so that Gil could examine her and tend to her multiple wounds. She lay almost folded at the bottom of the chair in the small box-like compartment meant for feet. She was leaning up on her elbows, so that she could see. Her long black hair was carefully combed and tied to the side with a string. She wore a smile that adorned her beautiful face.

When we first learned of her, her father had come to the Tree of Life seeking help for his daughter who lay at home on plastic feed bags in the dirt near their hut deep in the Savanna region of the bush. She was unable to sit up, unable to crawl, and had deteriorated into a lifeless form, attracting flies that landed and fed on the wounds of her lower body. She lay in her own feces and urine most of the time as keeping her clean without running water was a near impossible task for her family.

We drove our vehicle to their home through the paths of the jungle and found her just as her father had described. It was one of the first times that I had no immediate plan or vision of how we could help this child in this location and have it be more than a temporary fix.

My dear friend Gil, who is our amazing and creative wound care nurse, our pediatrician Jeri, and I tended to her wounds. Gil cleaned the sores that had grown to cover most of her buttocks and hips, and was slowly eating away what little flesh that she had. She was cleaned, dressed, ointment applied and provided with months of bandages and treatment supplies. It still wasn't enough, however, h to improve her life to a level greater than suffering.

We ordered a wheelchair when we got back into town the next day and had our driver deliver it to her. It was this chair that, for the first time in years, would make her mobile, and placed in a vertical position off the ground and out of the dirt.

Now years later, she returned to us, in the very chair that we had given her, and thanked us. Our dear Gil and Jane Vance, amazing artist from Virginia Tech, tended to Skameezie's needs. They lifted her from her box of confinement, and after cleaning it and making new pads to protect her body, Jane painted African animals in various colors surround the exterior and interior of her transportation device.

While removing the soiled and worn blankets they came across a tiny mirror about the size of a quarter - edges worn and smoothed over time. It was her only personal item that she coveted. The tiny mirror allowed this beautiful teenage girl to groom herself, and feel attractive. Gil, in her ways of wisdom, asked to trade the tiny worn mirror for a compact complete with a round mirror that she retrieved from her day pack. The trade was a good one. Skameezie was thrilled to have such a wonderful and unobtainable item, and so was Gil. The tiny worn mirror was given to Jane at the end of the day as a gift. It was her birthday, and she had spent it under the Tree of Life, deep in the bush of Africa.

Thou Shall Not Steal... Even a Little

We knew that something was going on and that greed was now in control. Theft, deceit, and corruption were the driving force and it had been going on for months behind our back, and right under our noses. Money was being made, and deposited into private accounts. False receipts were created for new materials when used items were actually being purchased. Cash flow was underground and certain people were getting rich, while workers were not getting paid. Anger grew fast in the village, as a sand business thrived at our expense.

Part of the land settlement included a large sand pit to the west of our property, bordering the entire back side. On its own, it looks like a large lake, that at one time, could hold an abundance of fish and be a water source for a community that had none.

The pit was now a large crater, vast and full of sand, the type that makes great cement, and sells like hot cakes in a community that builds their houses from homemade blocks.

No activity could ever be seen when we were in country, and no one knew anything about it when asked. The pit grew in size, but no one knew how or when.

"I'm flying over there this time unannounced. I don't want them to know we are coming and will need to stay that way. I want to see this business in action and then take action of our own," I said to Elijah, an OMNI's board member.

We determined that we needed to be there in person to handle this problem. We flew to Zambia, a quick twenty-three-hour flight. Time passes quickly I always say, with six meals and seven movies later, you are there. I changed into a business dress before landing and put on high heels. If I am going to fire him, it will be as professional and this time with some style. This was another mission that Scott needed to assist me with as I did not want to go alone.

He agreed.

According to Zambian culture, women were to be held accountable for many things - coming in unannounced and firing someone wasn't one of them. If you were to ask what the gender role of a woman was in Zambia, it would be to provide family care, and increase the number of people in their families. She must attend to daily household chores and to be "a wife" meaning she is humble and respectful to her husband. A woman in Zambia must be quiet and submissive to her husband.

Even though I am not a Zambian woman, I respect the culture that I found myself in, however, being in a leadership position and president of an organization whose sole purpose is to provide health care, education to all children, boys or girls, and provide community development, I had to stick to my guns and protect what we had established in this country, so that the children would be empowered through education and good health. Gender for me was not an issue in this case; I was respectful and very much aware of this cultural norm.

The plan was to have Felton meet in our attorney's office to receive an international call from the executive board about a random topic to peek his interest to drive into town. We arrived and were escorted to the second floor of a shop in downtown Ndola then into the attorney's back office. The office was quite bare; pictures hung near the ceiling, and never at eye level. *Odd*, I thought.

The outer office was reserved for clients waiting for their appointment of which Felton was just about to approach the scheduled time.

"You can't come into the country unannounced!" he hollered the moment he spotted us. "What are you doing here? You can't do this to me."

"Have a seat" said the attorney. "You remember Karen and Elijah and I'm sure you know Scott as well. Let's talk." The tension in the room was palpable and even though I felt we had the upper hand in the situation, my heart pounded.

Words flew across the room with the combining force of indignation and attempts of survival of a trapped animal. The law was read, clarification was made, and warnings were verbalized to make sure that Felton clearly understood what he was getting himself into. His answers to the attorney's questions about his involvement with missing funds and payments were ambiguous at best.

Instructions to give up the keys to the property, vehicles, and laptops were presented. To our surprise, and to perhaps his own, he got up and left the room without returning anything. A silence hung in the air as we witnessed his rapid exit from the meeting room. It was clear that the next step in this confrontation was necessary.

According to the penal code in Zambia: If the thing stolen is a vehicle the offender is liable to imprisonment for fourteen years.

Having been to several of the jails in Zambia with Elijah, praying for prisoners and also accompanying others who have stolen to reap the reward of their theft, it is a place clearly that you do not want to find yourself in...ever. Communicable diseases proliferate and come free with admission. Prolonged imprisonment is usually a death sentence in itself.

The following diet is clearly stated in the penal code book, however, family bears the responsibility to bring the diet to the prisoner. If no family is available, the time in prison is punishment beyond what we can imagine.

PENAL DIET: DAILY ISSUE

Maize meal . . . . .454 grams
or Millet meal . . . . .454 grams
or Bread . . . . .454 grams
Salt (iodized if possible) . . . . 7 grams
Unlimited water

The Ndola Central Police was just down the street and conveniently located near the center of town. The four level poorly painted building houses offices of the local police and the district chief of police, whose office resides at the very top of the aging structure. Since there are no elevators, you get to meet most everyone in the building as you ascend the stairs to the top. You stay to the left, something I have to remind myself of when in country, just as you do when you drive on any road in the country. Once on the 4th floor, you pass the office of the inspector, and enter the outer office of the chief of police.

"May I help you," she asked as we entered the secretary's office.

"Yes, we're here to see the chief, please," I said.

"I'll let him know you are here." Her cell phone acted as the inner office line, directly linking her to her boss who was concealed behind the closed wooden door. "He said you can go in."

We passed waiting clients, much to their surprise and ours.

"Karen, Elijah, how are you? What brings you to Zambia and more importantly to my office today?"

We had become friends or at least respected acquaintances over the past couple of years, and his hospitality and willingness to help right now was welcoming and fortuitous.

Our invitation to enter his office was met with mutual respect, and graciousness for being allowed sit on his right. The chair was pleasantly overstuffed and was large enough to line three walls of the office. Sofas and chairs such as these can be purchased along the roadside on the way to Kitwe. Furniture made of a variety of colors and fabrics adorn the roads for passengers and walkers to see. Their colors slowly fade in the sun and take on the dust that accumulates with each passing car.

A picture of the president hung near the top of the wall close to the ceiling. I acknowledged in my mind the pattern of locations for pictures as we were in the middle of this drama.

"I need your help on a situation with an employee who has refused to hand over the property keys, and has left with keys to two of our vehicles. We have reason to believe he is also involved in a large undercover sand business, stealing from our organization."

I could see that the chief was interested in our situation on several levels. "Of course, Karen, I can help you with that. I am sure you are aware of the laws here in Zambia."

I knew that theft of an automobile was serious, and in some cases could mean life in prison. The sand business was a whole other matter.

"It's already been a busy morning here, as you can see." He caught me looking down at a blue, soiled suitcase, just in front of his desk. The inexpensive flimsy excuse for a piece of luggage was slightly opened with contents waiting to overflow the cheap zipper that held it together. "Caught this guy this morning at the bus stop near the market. He was transferring these elephant tusks from Tanzania to South Africa for sale. As you know, the possession and sale of ivory is highly illegal. The poor guy was just the runner, but will take the punishment for the man who hired him." *Only in Africa would we be having this conversation,* I thought.

"Down the hall, we have a prisoner who is in the toilet room until he passes the balloon full of drugs that he swallowed when we arrested him. He'll wait until it passes or ruptures and in that case, he'll probably die of an overdose," the chief continued. "So I'm glad that you caught me early in the day before it got real busy."

We were in the presence of authority who dealt with corruption, stupidity, and criminal behavior on a daily basis. This was his "Monday morning at work." And he still had four more day's work ahead of him. The city should be grateful for his dedication to rid the area of these guys.

I was grateful for his support and his endorsement to allow us to state our case before him. The day could have been totally different if we were not given his time or attention. OMNI's past stellar reputation in the country and our work had preceded us. My hard work and care of the poor here was being endorsed by his full support.

Back to auto theft...the explanation was short, and the response was shockingly swift. He picked up his cell phone and called down to the main floor where the police officers waited for assignments. "I want three armed men, plain clothed, and a car." He waited. "We are going after a man wanted in auto theft." Pause. "Yes, now..." He hung up. "They will be right down," he said to me.

As we descended the three stories of steps, greeting other officers along the way and arrived on the main floor, we could hear the sound of rifles being loaded, chambers of AK47s being pulled back, and bullets inserted. Click...click. The men behind the counter were going into action and we were across the worn wooden intake station witnessing it. Serious action was being taken and we were right in the middle of it.

A few people waiting on the worn wooden bench just inside the door watched as the drama unfolded before all of our eyes.

Scott turned to me and said, "You didn't tell me that anyone was going to be killed on this trip!"

"They won't be," I said. Or at least I don't think so.

This was really happening, and it suddenly felt like we were transported into a live action movie. No one knew the rest of the script, but we were going along with it just the same.

The three armed officers dressed in old t-shirts, shorts, and various alterations of the same theme went ahead of us and got into a little white, beat up vehicle that clearly was the perfect cover for an undercover operation. We climbed into Elijah's car that had been parked in front of the police station since we arrived and kept our eyes on the undercover car as it pulled away from the police station.

I had a few concerns - one, being worried if the beat up vehicle that the police climbed into had the capability of doing a chase if needed; two, worried if we or someone would be shot. There was little time for more than that as we sped off after them. We traveled down the side streets just leaving enough space between us to not draw suspicion.

Interestingly enough, Felton, our guy on the run, had called in the morning to ask if we would meet him at the labor office. I believe that he thought if he was going to get fired, he would try and get some money from us for not giving notice. His plan was to have the labor office reprimand us and he would go free having had some retribution for the inconvenience.

In a tense and guarded phone conversation we said that we would meet him to talk, fully knowing that we were sending in the cavalry in our place. Imagine that, stealing vehicles, land and embezzling, and he wants back pay and a meeting with a government office! *Maybe we could even give him a going away party and a watch,* I thought.

We followed the police, keeping a safe distance, and parked a block away from the white car carrying the armed police. There was Felton, on the corner of an abandoned lot, next to the labor office, looking in all directions and occasionally over his shoulder. I slid down in my seat, as this little blond girl from the U.S. was probably noticeable even from a distance.

Scott was in the back and in a tone of disbelief, said, "I think this is where the bullets are going to fly."

I didn't respond, but thought he might be correct.

As always, Elijah was quite cool through this, and was actually pleased at our progress and the fact that we were in the middle of a sting that we had initiated. This isn't quite what I had in mind when I started medical missions for the poor, yet it was a part of the whole process. It did feel like we were deeper into this movie and weren't getting out very soon.

It was probably only a few minutes, but it seemed like a long time. Felton was leaning into the car appearing to give the apparently poor lost people inside directions. That's all that they needed. The two police, one from the front and one from the back, jumped out, cuffed him, and guided him into the back seat of the car. They had him, and now we would, again, for the second time in twenty-four hours, make a surprise appearance in front of our man Felton.

We ascended the four flights taking two steps at a time, still concentrating on staying to the left, so that we could get to the chief's office before the new prisoner arrived. Back to the sofa chair just to the right of the chief, the blue suitcase full of ivory still present, and some poor soul still locked in the bathroom awaiting his fate.

It was pitiful, seeing Felton like that. His hands behind him, cuffed, and a police officer on either side. He was escorted in and told to sit in a chair to the chief's left, near the open windows. The windows had cracks in the panes and one was even patched with layers of tape.

The chief's tone this time was of complete authority - no one in their right mind would challenge. The chief asked a few questions and then ordered Felton to stand up and to walk over to me and return the keys to our property. He complied, however, had the audacity to let some resemblance of contempt show through. Now that the keys to the vehicles had been returned, I still wondered where the vehicles were.

The next turn of events was almost comical and when we thought about it knew we couldn't even make it up. The chief told us that a vehicle showed up in the police parking lot and that it was locked and matched the one we were missing. The morning shift of police found it in their lot and wrote up a ticket for a parking violation. Imagine parking in the police lot without permission, and hiding a stolen vehicle in full view of the police! Felton had planned it so that the police would be looking everywhere but in their own back yard for our car, and he could now form an alibi that he was merely trying to return it and park it in a safe place. Brilliant! But, it didn't work as well as he planned. It was still theft and he was still under arrest.

The chief continued his gracious hospitality to us that day by loaning us two of the armed guards to drive our stolen vehicle and Felton, still in tow to our property. Once there we promptly loaded up all of his personal items, confiscated our laptop and records, and escorted him back to his home with instructions to never set foot on our property again.

The first olive branch was offered by agreeing to his release of a prison sentence. I had grown to like Felton over the years of his employment with us. He was always a personal kind of guy, polite, energetic, and possessed a good sense of humor. I had met his wife several times and their children and they seemed to be a close, involved family.

I didn't want to see him die in a horrible African prison, but I also knew he was done. He had lied and stolen from us for months. The bank account was missing funds, and there never seemed to enough money after I wired it to our business account to pay for what we had budgeted for. "Chapwa," as they say in their Bemba language. "It is finished." He and his sand business had some explaining to do.

Three years later, I received an e-mail from Felton's wife. He had suffered a severe stroke and was bedridden. His wife went on to explain that he wanted me to know of his situation, and that he was sorry for what he had done. I responded with prayers for healing and well wishes to the family.

From time to time, I get an e-mail from Felton telling me that he is improving and that his children are all in higher education and doing well. Although my trust in him was gone, the memories of our time spent caring for the vulnerable children remained.

Throughout the years, I have feared a few situations in life. My biggest fear, however, is the awareness of betrayal from those that I trusted within an understood inner circle of friends and family. Evil within had violated my sense of security, and heightened my awareness from that point on.

Our work week continued with damage control and work to be done at the OMNI site. Each day was different from the last and each day had its unique earmarks as Africa always does. We were traveling back from the OMNI school late at night around twenty hours and we came to a stop sign just to the right of the large cemetery.

It was a four way stop and to our left was a truck pulling an open bed trailer. Peering from the back of the truck, and many feet higher than the roof, was a giraffe. He was clearly out of context, out of place and unexpected. He looked left and right, we did as well, and we proceeded, moving past this amazing creature being transported from who knows where, and hopefully to someplace that was conducive to his species. It was Africa, it was nighttime, and nothing surprised me.

It was 2009, and shortly after Elijah left for the airport to fly back to the U.S., I contracted malaria. It came upon me suddenly and without warning. I was walking down the street of Ndola and felt a severe and intense headache developing. Within a few minutes, my strength drained from me and my joints, especially my knees, ankles, and back developed pain that felt like I had fractures in all joints. The ground started to roll under my strides and I felt faint. Malaria has an alias in Africa called "Bone breaking disease." The title was correctly named.

I am not one to complain or draw attention for aches or pains, but this was different. In my mind, I thought that if I could only get to the pharmacy and sit outside on a bench, and I could seek help from my pharmacist friend who owned the large company. The bench became my new goal that day. I could barely make it, but I did. I did not make it back inside. That was a distance that I could not muster up enough strength to accomplish. I needed to get to the car now and lay down. My assessment was simple - I had malaria and it was a very strong case.

I had to tell Scott, who was walking with me, about my assumptions. Elijah was leaving for the airport shortly to head back to the States so he was off gathering his bags to prepare for the flight. He returned with our car and found me now slumped to one side unable to sit up.

"I hate to leave you like this," Elijah said.

But he did.

I hoped for a moment he could stay and help but it was clear that he had an agenda to keep and that did not include my welfare. He left me and Scott there and we would have to fend for ourselves. We did but it was not easy. It was the most challenging thing I have done in my life…

As my body went limp and with no physical energy, all I could think of was the mission that needed to be cared for - my family at home and that Scott was with me. Thank God for Scott. He was the most capable person to have with me and I would eventually owe my life to him. He was there for me once again.

By the time we got back to the lodge, I could barely walk, and lay on the bed to see if it would pass. Well that was delusional all by itself. By nightfall, fever, and nausea had set in, and all symptoms were increasing. I knew that I was in trouble, and feared going to the local hospital, having taken patients there before. The standards were not conducive to survival, and many people once admitted, did not leave on their own power. As the number one killer on the continent, too many people lost their lives to this dangerous disease.

The front desk suggested going to a private clinic run by a physician from Cuba who had come here to earn a living. The lady gave us the street address, and a general location of the facility. By now, darkness had settled in and it would be hours before the sun rose. Roads had no street signs or lamp posts and we were at the mercy of God and our driver to get to this clinic.

The burgundy car had a new alarm system put in again, and as luck would have it, or lack of it, it would not open. Our driver and Scott worked feverishly trying to get it open as I lay down on the grass, resting my head on a large rock near the driveway entrance. It was hard and cold, but my body could not hold it or me up. The rock was my pillow and I really didn't care.

We could not wait any longer, and I heard the sounds of broken glass as they broke through the back window with a large flashlight. Scott crawled in through the opening and opened up the car so that I could be helped in. We drove, and drove in what seemed like forever. I was so sick and getting worse as time went on. I tilted to the left and went horizontal at least from my waist up on the seat of the car. Scott kept vigil, not overly attentive as that is not his style, but concerned none the less.

We arrived at 11:45 p.m. at a clinic only to find that it had closed. Time seemed to be against us. We left and went on to the clinic that we had originally been trying to find. It was clean, small, and seemed to be capable of taking care of my needs. The nurse on call was resting behind the desk as the tiny waiting room was empty. She took my blood pressure, noting it was low, took my temperature and noted that it was 102 degrees.

The next step was to do a blood test, with a finger prick to test for malaria. I heard Scott ask if the needle was new and not used. I didn't really care at this point as I felt too weak to worry about any tests, however, appreciated his keen sense of medical asepsis. I saw the blood test placed in a metal bowl on a tray near my head.

In fifteen minutes, the test came back positive. From that point, the nurse escorted me into a small bathroom to give a urine sample. I wasn't sure that I could make it to provide what they needed, but she helped me and stayed with me. The urine test that she requested showed blood in the urine indicating kidney involvement at an early stage in this disease. I knew that malaria was the number one killer in the continent, and feared for my life and recovery.

I was given a small yellow and red box that contained Co-Arinate and had the instructions written in English on one end and a foreign language on the other. It had been manufactured in Nairobi, Kenya, and was the current drug of choice for malaria. On the insert wrapped around the three large pills, the instructions read:

"Malaria is caused by Plasmodium falciparum, is serious, life threatening disease and requires a complete cure." There were three more pages of instructions, contraindications, and warnings. My instructions were to take 1 tab daily, in addition to Cipro a very powerful antibiotic, 1000mg. daily for the kidney involvement.

The drive back to the lodge was worse than the drive to the clinic, as I wasn't' sure I could make the trip. Once back in my room, the fever came and went, so did the vomiting and diarrhea, and I spent the rest of the night trying to cool down on the cold tile floor that covered the small bathroom. I had very little strength left, and I seemed to get worse instead of better.

The next morning, I could barely drink water, and I knew I was getting dehydrated - weaker by the minute. The combination of the Cipro and Co-Arinate were now causing cardiotoxicity, and I felt like someone was standing on my chest. I was sure that this was how I was going to die, as many do here.

I was rushed back to the clinic and within a few minutes the doctor from Cuba arrived, examined me then made a startling announcement to Scott. "Malaria is my bread and butter so to speak," he boasted. "Fifty percent of the people who get malaria recover and fifty percent die. She is in the percentage that will not make it. I think that she has cerebral malaria and should be put on IV quinine."

I told Scott to call home back in the U.S. and tell them what was going on. The last thing that I wanted was to be put on an IV drip here, knowing that patients who are on this treatment hallucinate and become often times unconscious.

"No, I would rather go back to the lodge and tough it out. No quinine," I said in a weak voice.

"She is not making any sense, and if she checks out, it will be against my instructions and I will not treat her again," he proclaimed as I lay on the gurney, unable to lift my head or arms.

The phone conversation between Scott and my husband back in the U.S. was interesting, even from the one side that I could hear. "She isn't making sense, and she won't let them start the IV," Scott said. "It doesn't look good on this end," he concluded.

I remember being assisted, and perhaps more accurately loaded into the back seat of our SUV in the early hours of October. 18, 2009. My understanding of the situation was that I would not make it home, but I would not die in a Cuban clinic strapped to a gurney hallucinating secondary to IV quinine. This felt like the end.

We drove back to the lodge and I lay on the bathroom floor that night vacillating between fever and chills, nausea, and extreme lethargy. Morning finally came.

There is a saying in Africa, "No matter how long the night, morning will come."

I was grateful.

"Scott, I need you to take over OMNI and get this work done," I said. It was the only thing that I could think of to keep the mission going. Scott took in all that I had asked and with my assistant on the ground, they left for the day to buy food, supplies and conduct necessary chores to keep the children of OMNI School well fed and cared for.

I needed to get home and see Gil. I needed to get home and support my dear friend. I needed to get out of Africa alive.

What was even more devastating was the evil and heinous crime that had taken place back in Virginia just hours before. I was lying on the bed of the lodge, unable to reach the cell phone as it rang. *I will call them back, when I have the strength*, I thought.

Less than an hour later, I reached for the phone and heard the voice of my best friend. "Karen, we have a family emergency here. I don't want to bother you while you are in Africa, but Morgan is missing."

I called Gil back on the international cell phone going through all of the call numbers, and international codes. Gilberte Harrington was the mother of Morgan Danna Harrington, who went missing the night before from John Paul Jones Arena on October 17, 2009, while attending a Metallica concert in Charlottesville, Virginia. It was a surreal. I needed to be with Gil, and could not be there. I thought I would not make it off this continent. Morgan was missing, unheard of, and already not sounding good. *She could not be missing*, I thought. It's a nightmare, and I need to wake up.

It was October 25 when Scott and I landed in Washington, DC. The flight home was a challenge. I was fortunate to find three seats unoccupied on the flight and was able to lie horizontal for most of the time. I felt too weak to do much less. The floor despite being off limits to airline passengers was my second option. I drank as much water as I could and advanced to ginger ale. Food was of no interest to me.

We drove an hour to Scott's apartment, which again seemed a long way away. I had to rest before I could gather up enough energy so that I could shower and try to regroup. I had lost a fair amount of weight and was dehydrated, but was determined to make it to the breakfast just one block away. I guess that there was no food in his apartment, but I wondered why we could not have just had some brought in.

The walk there took all of my energy, and my heart pounded like crazy. Each step felt like I had cement shoes on and was carrying weights on my arms. The skin on my face felt too heavy for my head to carry. I was weak but grateful to have made it home. I needed to go and see my dear friends who were in crises with the disappearance of their most precious Morgan. Prayers were constant for Morgan and her family.

We drove from DC to Roanoke, a four hour plus ride on a good day and went directly to their home. I remember focusing all of my strength to walk down their brick path to the front door, and then embraced Gil and Dan with what energy I had left.

We went into their living room, and they explained the mystery and the agony of Morgan's disappearance, the circumstances of the event, and their despair. I could only lie on their sofa and try to imagine what these wonderful people were trying to deal with. For them, the nightmare had just begun. I vowed to do everything that I could for my best friend to help her through this nightmare. How could it ever be enough? No amount of support could bring her back, but I vowed to be there for Gil every day. Their precious beautiful daughter was missing and most likely would not be coming home again.

Rumors and actual verbalizations from the board admitted that they thought I would never return to Africa. The speculation was that I would resign from being president of OMNI and curl up somewhere trying to feel sorry for myself or something of that nature.

I'm not an equestrian, but I do remember that someone once said, " If you fall of the horse, get up and ride again soon." Or something like that.

A month later, my family attended a massive search for Morgan in Charlottesville along with 1,200 other volunteers from all over the state. The search lasted three days and included mounted search teams on horseback, K9 units and ground teams. I had the opportunity to be assigned as field support for one of the K9 units from Virginia assigned to the point last seen.

It was after that search that I decided to join a K9 unit, hire a trainer and get a dog to honor Morgan. Savanna, a beautiful golden retriever the color of the great Savanna in Africa became my search partner and opened the door to SAR work and many more years of valuable form of service. Savanna was the first of three working dogs that I run, train, and own in search of the missing.

We are nationally certified and dedicated to search for the missing to bring them home to their families. After Savanna, Haley, and Tango also search in her name.

Morgan's remains were discovered on January 26, 2010, about ten miles from the arena in a remote area of a large private farm. At that time her abductor and murderer remained at large. The days, months, and years for Dan and Gil have been dedicated to working long and hard days and night to bring justice for Morgan. Their love for her is endless as they remember their daughter with positive and productive measures to trump the evil with good. They are doing just that and have successfully created the Help Save the Next Girl foundation in her memory.

On December 1, 2010 the Morgan Harrington Educational Wing was officially opened on the campus of the OMNI Village by Dr. Maureen Mwanawasa, the former First Lady of Zambia. It was an honor to be hosting such an event and for the first time in almost two years, our school had an even greater purpose that before. Our children from the Village of George, coming from the poorest of poor families, would enter the hallowed doors of Morgan's School. Her dream was to become a school teacher, and this building was constructed to honor her life and her desire to educate children.

Children who pass through the doors of Morgan's School struggle through life with little or nothing. Attending the school gives them a future and hope. Upon our annual home visits, we record the profiles of each child and their living conditions. While the homes are generally clean and well kept, there are little to no personal belongings. There is little if any furniture, little in the way of clothes, and only a few pots, pans, or dishes. Rainy season is damaging to these barren homes and leaves many of them with leaky roofs, where the elephant grass, pieces of scrap plastic and tin don't meet.

Cooking is usually done outside over an open fire and consists of a corn based meal, greens that grow in the fields, kapenta (dried fish) supplemented by rats and mice which have been trapped and killed.

Birds often succumb to the sling shots that the children have and help to supplement the meal.

Age is irrelevant and really not very much of any importance here. Not everyone knows the year that they were born, and few know the month. Almost no one knows the actual date. It's just not important. What is important is that you are here, and still alive. Time doesn't matter either. It is the event that matters and the fact that you are there even if you are hours or days late! It makes more sense to me now that I am in this space in my life. What you wear is of the lowest on this list of needs. I confess that I have wasted too much time in my life worrying if what I had on was the right thing to wear or looked "Ok" for the occasion. Time wasted for sure. Shelter of any kind is paramount to survival. Health care is a deal breaker for most.

Families here consist of the children and the adults, and not all children are born to the parents, with the adults taking in other relatives' children due to illness, death, or divorce. Some parents have simply left their children behind, succumbing to the extreme pressure of raising them. Lack of income and alcoholism play a significant factor in everyone's lives.

The days that the children do not come to our school, is usually a day at home with little or no food. Food at the school has become a means of sustaining many lives here, focusing on the needs of the children first.

James lives with his aunt and his two cousins. His aunt is mentally challenged and is unmarried - divorced. Her source of income is to brew and sell the local beer, kachasu. There are five other children living in the house and all of them suffer from headaches, seasonal malaria, and diarrhea. Veronica who is eleven and living in the house walks to the OMNI School every day. She wants to be a nurse someday and draws on scraps of paper as her hobby. There is not enough food in the home, so the meals served at OMNI every day has helped to save her life.

Oliver, Dorris, and Rachael are double orphans, living with their widowed grandmother. Their two cousins - seven and ten - recently came to live her also when both of their parents tested positive for HIV/AIDS. Oliver is ten and wants to be a pilot, and Dorris wants to be a nurse and hopes someday to have a doll. Rachael is twelve and in third grade. She wants to be a policewoman when she is done with school. Their grandmother earns a little bit of money by selling mulembwe, Zambian okra which grows wild in the bush. They all eat one meal a day in the evening, and attend church in George on Sunday together.

Collins, Roger, and Emma are part of a family with one father and three wives. There are twenty-five children in all ranging in age from twenty-six to three years. Fortunately, the father is a farmer and has some pigs, goats, and chickens. Not all children go to school, but they feel blessed to have one meal a day. Money is very tight and resources are few.

Nathan lives just down the main dirt road and to the left going down a few houses. He wants to be a doctor when he grows up and definitely has the intelligence to do so. He lives with his mother and father and is one of eight children. Nathan's father burns wood to create charcoal that can be sold on the roadside for a heat source. When we first met Nathan several years ago, he limped into the clinic using a tree limb, holding up the shriveled leg on his left side. He had malaria when he was a small child and originally both legs were paralyzed. After some physical therapy at the Children's Hospital in town, he fortunately regained use of one of his legs. He was denied surgery on his affected leg since he had one that did function. OMNI fitted him for crutches and purchased special shoes that provide a lift on the left side.

With money so very scarce and the family being large, we brought food to him home on one occasion while I was there. The only thing cooking that night on the fire was greens and water. Nathan was handed a large bag of fresh bread. He reached into the bag and took out a large piece which I thought would go directly into his mouth. He gave it to his small brother and waited until he finished his share. Nathan was a thin and frail, and had a heart bigger than we knew. OMNI now sends food to his family every month to support his family.

Sarah wants to be a nurse and likes to read now that she has attended school. There are twelve children in the family, including four sets of twins -two died from malaria, one died from having measles, and one died of anemia. Her father is a tailor and makes some money through his work, but suffers from mental problems. He has to be restrained when he becomes aggressive and has mad fits. The family however has little complaints when asked except for malaria and coughing. The school has been a blessing to the family in general.

The social histories are all similar in that poverty and lack of clean water, proper shelter, clothing, unite them. The OMNI School, especially Morgan wing represents hope and a brighter future. It is the ray of hope in the middle of absolute poverty and despair.

Outside of the Morgan Harrington Educational building, grows the most beautiful pink rose bush that I have ever seen. It grows in the very spot where some of her ashes were lovingly spread by her mother shortly after her remains were found. Morgan's rose blooms and reflects the beauty of a beautiful young woman, stolen without permission well before her time. You have graced the land that no one deemed as valuable and is now valuable to many, especially the children who if they knew you would love you.

The beauty of this school is that OMNI interviews over one hundred extremely impoverished children for only thirty spots each year for the first grade. All children desperately want to attend as it is their only hope for a future. We can only choose one third as this is all of the space and resources that we have. It is as heart breaking as it is to lose Morgan, to turn away children who would have been educated in her name simply because we don't have the space or the funds.

The thirty that are chosen are immediately given food, medicines if needed, a school uniform and a spot in life to excel. Morgan would have loved this! This small structure mirrors her aspirations in the world as an educator and as a humanitarian following closely in her loving mother's footsteps.

Her legacy lives on with every child that enters her doors and she is forever loved.

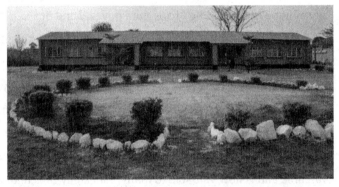

Morgan Harrington Educational Wing at the OMNI School

Baluba: Congolese Refugee Village

Our work led us to the village of Baluba - a Congolese refugee village whose people fled from the violence. They were safe for now. The village bordered northern Zambia, and contained an invisible border full of illegal crossings points. There were many people seeking a life free from violence, free from atrocities that maimed them, and free from death.

Each person fled with a tremendous amount of courage. There were spots where border patrol guards could not access, so mothers, daughters, fathers, sons, and their distant relatives were able to sneak through to freedom.

I couldn't help but wonder if they sought their freedom in the light of day or under the cover of darkness. *I should have asked them*, I thought. I needed to focus on why we were there and that they needed our help. They were brave to leave and desperate to live.

The dirt path leads straight into the center of the tiny village. Shanty homes dotted the area. Makeshift bars selling homebrewed alcohol surrounded by the early morning inebriated young men lined our path. Children with swollen empty bellies and snot running from their noses ran alongside the car. The adults stood in the background. Women were bathing babies in a pan of dirty water more than likely shared by previous siblings. Some were hanging clothes on the bushes to dry in the African sun. Most of the elderly never acknowledged our passing and stared tirelessly into nowhere as we drove by.

I had no idea where we would set up our clinic, but knew that we needed to be here.

We drove deeper into the collection of people and found the perfect spot - an uninhabited wooden structure painted green quite some time ago. There were no windows, no doors, and no floor, but it would suffice as a shelter and a form of crowd control. We parked our small bus, pulling behind an open bed trailer full of our duffels and

227

medical supplies. *Please dear God, keep us safe, and let me have what I need in our bags to treat this group of needy refugees.*

The line grew by two with each one we treated. Their medical needs consisted of infections, starvation, burns from brush fires, and more. No one in our clinic spoke Congolese and the Congolese did not speak English and it worked perfectly for this mission. We would make it work and take care of the multiple afflictions.

Very early on in the clinic, we had a need for wound care but had no sterile area to set it up. I looked down the dusty dirt road and saw the bars, the children, and the mass of humanity that needed help. Nothing looked like a resource for a clinical set up.

"Let's put a surgical drape on the hitch of the trailer," I said. It is off the ground, is near the bus, and will work just as well as anything we have."

My third son Daniel, who was approaching eighteen and his friend were happy to have direction and created a wound station that would easily stand up throughout the day's challenges. I looked over to them at one point and saw a woman lying on her side having her ear irrigated. Daniel used his innovative skills well and his idea of helping the woman from in front of the trailer was working. The hitch was our new wound station and was serving the purpose.

An opening in the west wall of the wooden structure served as my station. A small elderly woman with a gnarled hand was next in line. She placed her brown hand on the narrow ledge that divided us.

Immediately I saw that her middle finger was missing just below the knuckle. The stump was healed - indicating that the source of trauma had occurred sometime in the distant past. With a rapid assessment it was clear that she had no other needs but that of a missing finger. My eyes left her and scanned the crowd for anyone who could speak any English.

A man behind her stepped forward and gave me my answer.

A few months ago the woman had been struck on the hand by a cobra snake. Her finger eventually fell off after it died.

"Could we help her get her finger back?" Was what she wanted to know. I had him explain to her that there was no cure for the event that had taken her finger. We were creating our own medical care in a makeshift clinic, and things were just as God had expected. Compassion was there, the need was there, medicine was there, and we were willing to care. How could you start to explain this one to her? I can still see her hand on the ledge to this day.

We continued our travel back to Baluba, a village that other teams feared and excluded by the government because of their origination. I found their needs to be most challenging and as the years went on, found this to be the place that I longed to go. It was the most difficult clinic for our team - lacking order, lacking leadership, and lacking any support from the outside world. It was a perfect place for a Christian medical mobile clinic who wants to make a difference in the world. We have been there now for almost a decade.

I learned over the years that one person can change one person's life - forever...what a profound concept and revelation. The change can take place in a moment, or in a heartbeat. It doesn't take much except compassion and courage. We all have that in us and it costs nothing to give away.

Our team was now working on the main street of Baluba, a bombed-out in appearance gray cement "L" shaped one story building made by hand. The building was to be the community school, but the government did not support it and the refugees, now in the hundreds, had no money to provide for teachers or to keep it functioning. Windows made of thin glass inserted into steel rusty frames were broken and did not close properly. Doors were missing on a few rooms. Other doors were locked to protect the meager contents of a couple of broken desks within. There were about fifteen rooms and none of them were functional for a classroom. It reminded me of a Hotel 6 gone bad - abandoned and desolate.

The grounds were uneven hard dirt, laden by weeds that had been trampled by passing villagers time and time again. One tree on the grounds provided shade for the weary and for our vehicle if we could get a chance to have it parked for that long.

We stationed ourselves as a mobile unit with the pharmacy at the far end. It was the last stop in the line of care that we could provide. It had two windows for an RN at each station to pass out the medications and the instructions that would hopefully cure the disease or ailment that was afflicting the patient. It was the bottleneck of the clinic, where as a team, you would use your head lamp in the dark of night to fill the last 100 prescriptions of the day and scramble to put all evidence away of your medications into the duffels and place them safely on the bus before being mobbed or threatened.

Earlier in the day, a thin weary woman came into the line carry a small boy whose head appeared too big for his body. His arms were no larger around than two of my fingers. Hi cheekbones protruded from his thin face and seemed to hold up his sunken black eyes. Both mother and son seemed emaciated and worn beyond words from the life that they were enduring. A large scar on the middle of her forehead revealed the evidence of her survival of the wielding axe attack brought on by her alcoholic husband. In prison now, she was free to come to the clinic to seek help for her and her son. His siblings were left at home to fend for themselves, as they often are in this society.

We learned that their symptoms were that of weight loss, night sweats, loss of appetite, fever, chills, and more weight loss.

"Can we do a blood test to see if you have something going on that would cause these symptoms?" our lab person asked as he came closer. "And the baby, what is his name? Can we check his blood as well?"

"Peter," she said. He had desperation in his eyes and kept constant eye contact with his mother. The nonverbal language was deafening. They spoke to each other with a strong eye contact and void of words. His tiny thin fingers hung tightly onto the dirty worn collar on the shirt of his mother. His mother looked into his fearful eyes and without words said, "I know Peter, and I know that you are dying."

Both tested positive for HIV AIDS. Peter, had advanced disease and with his limited life on earth, already possessed the knowledge and sense of his demise. His large dark eyes were intensely focused on his mother as he struggled to stay with her. His body was failing him and so was the society that he lived in. He would soon become another statistic that veiled this continent.

Peter's mother had no means to care for him properly at home, and being ill herself gave us permission to place the failing toddler in a home for HIV positive babies just next to her village, and within walking distance. Babies there would be cared for in a loving manner by a Catholic church group out of Canada. They offered nourishment, clean clothes, and cribs that were provided by donors who wanted to help the tiny victims of this disease. Despite the love and care, Peter died two weeks into his stay at the Hope House.

The following year, Peter's mother came to the medical clinic we were conducting at the colorless cement block building in Baluba. Her appearance was very much like the year before - thin, distraught, and full of grief. I heard through people in the crowd that she was looking for me. When I scanned the mass of humanity before our clinic, I saw her standing under the only tree that gave shelter and shade. She was holding a fragile, cracked picture of Peter, which she pulled from her torn oversized shirt.

The cries and sounds that came from her when she saw me reminded me of an animal that had been injured or trapped in the woods - traumatized and begging for an escape. I knew her only as "Bana Peter", or the mother of Peter. I walked over to her and embraced this grown frail women with my arms open to hold her up. This allowed her to cry and express her loss with less effort as she had little else in her to give. Peter was dead, and she wanted to tell me without the benefit of interpretation of the language of how she felt.

I understood.

I heard her.

As a mother, my heart broke for her as I could feel her body physically react to her grief. She needed to connect with someone who had cared for and knew her son who had died far too young. I could see Peter's eyes as she wept. Haunting.

She eventually left the clinic with the worn picture placed next to her heart, and faded into the countryside. Her skin covered her frail body and was marked by multiple assaults and abuse. Her thin chest, ribs, and veins gave shape and bore the image of her son, close to her heart. She turned and walked away, back into the very village that would be her destination that day. I worried about her and thought perhaps that she may have eventually died of a broken heart before AIDS could claim her.

I have not seen her since.

Hundreds of people gathered under the tree where she had stopped and our clinic was hours from being complete.

A Carpentry of Miracles

The Salem Rotary Club invited me to attend their meeting held at noon in a large conference room. I was honored once again to attend and to be in the presence of such accomplished business men and women who donated their time to international and local causes that would benefit our communities globally - and at home. It was a meeting that I had been invited to before, and had actually been a guest speaker on many occasions.

They said that it was award day and that I would be receiving one of the awards.

The meeting was large with over 150 people in attendance. My name was called and to my surprise I was awarded the Paul Harris Fellow Award for international humanitarian efforts. The metal hung on a blue and yellow ribbon and the lapel pin that accompanied it was an honor and recognition to my work in Africa.

Later that afternoon while finishing up some paperwork in my office in Virginia, my phone rang.

"Hello?" I asked, half listening.

"I have heard about OMNI and have nowhere else to turn," said the man.

Our connection wasn't the greatest, but I could hear him none-the-less.

"Uh uh, how can I help you?" He had my attention.

"This is John and I am calling from Seeds of Hope in Zambia, Africa. I hope that you can help me."

One of the village teachers in the northeastern province of Zambia contacted John about a young boy named Anderson who needed his help. The boy was born with bilateral congenital abnormalities of the feet, meaning that both feet were roughly sixteen inches long and proportionately wide. Anderson was a bright child that lived in a residential school setting for special needs children in a remote village near the Congo border in the north. His mother worked long hours in a field near their village home. She saved all of the money she could to pay for his education. The many miles between her home and the work field put her safety at risk daily.

Anderson was in extreme pain at all times and often hid in his room to shield himself from the ridicule that he received due to his infirmity. Getting to the classroom was a burden and he often times would not eat because walking to the school cafeteria was too painful. He was thin, depressed, and equally shy.

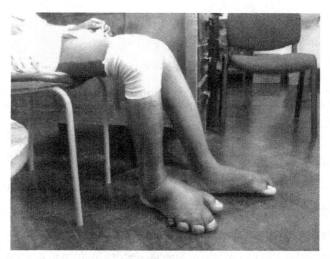

One of the teachers in his school even charged people to come and see Anderson's feet - as though he were a sideshow act in the circus. The teacher, of course, pocketed most of the money and gave Anderson a very small portion for his willingness to be on display.

Anderson learned quickly that the money, as little as it was, helped his mother. He also learned how to make more money from the little he had.

When the children of the school needed money for food during their school breaks, Anderson would loan a small amount to them, making them agree to not only return the loan, but to return it with a small amount of interest. The money that he earned was given to his mother - such was his life, filled with pain and humiliation.

"We have taken him to the capital and to the university hospital for an evaluation. They said that the only thing they could do for him

236

was to amputate above the knee on both legs," John said, his voice heavy.

My mind raced as I envisioned this young boy having both of his legs amputated and the physical and emotional trauma that he would have to endure because of it. Beyond that his likelihood for survival in an African village as an amputee would be extremely arduous and debilitating. I immediately recalled a middle aged man in one of our villages who we served who had both legs amputated following a road accident. His means of mobility was to scoot around the village on his bottom, using the knuckles of his hands to propel his body forward. His eyes were always at the level of passerby's knees, and were no higher than the wild dogs that roamed the countryside.

"Please don't let them amputate his legs!" I begged. "Let me see what I can do here and I will get back to you. I am hoping that we can find someone here that can help this young boy and save his legs if possible."

When I hung up the phone, I immediately called Dr. Charles Zelen, a surgical podiatrist in town who had also operated on Memory's foot a few years prior. He was the best that I knew in the region. We needed two miracles now, to save this one child.

"Hi, Dr. Chuck, I am going to need a big favor from you if you are willing," I said with caution.

"What do you have for me this time?" Dr. Chuck asked.

I tried to explain the condition of Anderson as quickly as I could - time was of the essence.

Faxes, e-mails, and more phone calls back and forth continued until we had a plan for this young man. Lewis Gale Hospital in Roanoke agreed to provide the hospital stay - a costly bill for the complicated surgery.

A medical visa was issued in Zambia for his entry into the U.S. almost immediately, as were shoes, which he owned none. Anderson was to stay at my home for his pre and post-op care, which was sure to extend into nine months. My being a medical professional, allotted him the ability to stay in a home rather than a hospital setting.

A Canada native from one of the local tribes made hand-sewn moccasins using elk hides that were lovingly lined with rabbit fur. John traced his large foot on a sheet of paper and sent it to her to use as a pattern. The moccasins were decorated with a teardrop and symbols of good fortune for this young man. The handmade shoes were his first and only pair of coverings that held his distorted feet. They would be the very items that would allow him permission to enter a commercial airplane and travel the 3,000 miles from Africa to Virginia. His courage was in place, and John traveled with Anderson to start his medical journey in the U.S.

Food, clothing, a home with heat, electricity, and running water was as new to him as his dramatic entrance to this country, stepping on the ground with one foot and pivoting to sit on the wheelchair that carried him into the airport.

I met him for the first time, and was determined that his stay would be as close to him having a second home as possible. It took courage to come here, not knowing what would lie ahead medically, personally, and spiritually. His faith in God allowed him to make the journey of a thousand steps toward his future.

X-rays, scans, blood work, and multiple doctor visits continued weekly for the next two months in preparation for his surgery. He became a part of our family, living in my daughter's old room on the main floor of our home. In two months, he ate, drank milk, took vitamins, learned English and gained over twenty pounds. His skinny shoulders started to fill out, and his face lost the hollowness in his cheeks. We made more shoes out of orthopedic slippers and duct tape. He began to make friends at church and within the community as I took him everywhere.

Anderson asked to be baptized at our church, as he felt before he went into such a serious surgery, his spiritual life needed to be in order. He was baptized by total immersion as requested, and the ceremony was done by our pastor who was also from Zambia. Anderson was happy that day and said that the only thing missing was his mother.

He loved my dogs, and they loved him. They seemed to sense that there was a medical challenge for him that required their attention, and often they laid on the floor next to him, which in turn gave him much needed comfort.

The day finally came for surgery, and the media, and friends gathered to watch this young boy face what would be a grueling six-hour reconstruction and reconfiguration of his left foot. Hemovac drains were placed inside the foot to drain the operative sites from where blood accumulated. Pain medication was administered via an infusion pump in an attempt to control the excruciating pain of the surgically-altered bones and muscles of his foot. Our pastor came and gave him communion in the hospital room and prayed over him as his pain was near unbearable.

After four days, Anderson was allowed to come home. I loaded him in the back of my SUV surrounded by pillows with his foot elevated. Before heading home, he asked to stop at a fast-food chain for a large drink and a big juicy cheeseburger - a good sign of recovery.

Three months went by with nursing care in our home, 6 a.m. weekly dressing changes at the doctor's office, and numerous long talks encouraging his compliance with his care, and his willingness to consider the next surgery on his right foot. Each and every single day Gil, my dear friend, would meet us in the parking lot of the hospital just shortly after 6 a.m. to support the dressing changes, and always gave encouragement and often times a gift for Anderson to cheer him up. She documented every office visit on her camera and was there the morning of his surgeries, going into the pre-operative suite before the nurse wheeled Anderson to the operating room. I needed to see her just as much as Anderson needed to see her - we were a team. It was not an easy journey for Anderson, or for anyone who gave all we had to save this young boy's legs *and* his life.

Post operatively the incisions were stressed from the massive amount of swelling in his foot, and multiple wound care sessions to maintain a sterile site, along with antibiotics were given to keep the site from getting infected. It was difficult to keep Anderson's spirits up with the healing process, which included painful dressing changes, but each day, he did it.

Four months after the first surgery with the assistance of a walker, Anderson made his first step on his new foot. Now it was time for the second surgery and decisions had to be made on the extent and the risks involved.

After a great deal of consultation and more tests, we decided to do a partial amputation of the right foot, as the vascular anomalies and the bones were beyond what could be done similar to the left foot.

Again, the surgery lasted almost seven hours, and the massive irregular appendage was given shape and sculptured with amazingly skilled hands of Dr. Charles Zelen, head of Roanoke Foot and Ankle Associates.

He was an artist in the operative field and an angel here on earth with all his patients. For Anderson - the cost was $0. I am forever grateful to Dr. Zelen.

As the physical healing took place, we also provided care for the emotional healing needed for Anderson to return to Africa. Anderson not only transformed physically, but mentally as well. The progress, although served bits at a time, were great. Pain comes quickly at an instant. Healing can take a lifetime.

Watching Anderson shed his emotionally protective shell was wondrous for us all. We took him everywhere with us. He went to church with me in a wheelchair, and eventually on crutches. Each time people greeted him and commented on his progress. Each interaction was like a powerful vitamin to boost his confidence and his inner strength.

I took him with me to my K9 lessons for the search and rescue team. He told me how much people liked him and how great it was to see him. His smile broadened and his personality bloomed.

I bought him new clothes, and provided him books and educational materials, which were soaked up like a dry cloth in water.

Gil and her husband bought Anderson a laptop and on one of his weekend stays with them, taught him how to use it. He loved to learn and craved ways to better himself. He seemed to enjoy the new technology. He read books we had in the basement that were doing nothing but gathering dust.

Members in our church and community were most gracious to this young man and came and took him out to the movies, lunch, dinner, church events, and just plain exposure to everyday life. Anderson grew and matured with confidence and a new revelation of acceptance. His feet were no longer the focus. He was the focus and people liked him as he was.

Three months later, several skin grafts, multiple office visits, home dressing changes, and many prayers, Anderson was ready to fly back to Zambia - this time walking on his two new feet and wearing size 15 shoes. His favorites were the ones with the check on the side - he said it made him look just like the other guys his age.

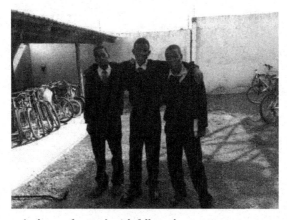

Anderson (center) with fellow classmates.

Anderson went on to finish his high school education and was accepted into a college in the capital of Zambia. Another life saved, and another child lifted to allow him to reach his greatest potential in life.

Our medical team returned to Zambia that following summer and Anderson came to the clinic one day to work as our interpreter. "I need to give back," he said. "I want to help those who are not as fortunate as I am." His smile radiated.

Within the medical clinic, Anderson was helping in pharmacy by packing vitamins and filling prescriptions. At mid-point in the day, he came forward and served as my interpreter as I handed out lifesaving medications to the waiting patients. With the help of God, Anderson came full circle.

"Song bird! Fly, fly away."

For most of the team on our next trip to Zambia, it was their first trip to there, and their first to Africa. For me it was my thirty-ninth trip and just another flight home to the country that I love. I had left for Africa with well wishes from my children and the absence of any spousal support. The day before my departure, I saw a sticky note on the counter. It was from my husband. On it he told me that he had left and was not coming home. I was determined to be strong and to continue onto Africa to do the work that was waiting for me.

After the twenty-three-hour flight, and two days after leaving the comforts of our home, and thoroughly exhausted, my next hurdle was to pass through customs and not be arrested or detained.

This has been going on for fifteen years, despite my intense attention to every detail of the packing of medications and the creation of the manifest.

Once inside the small quonset that serves as the international airport into Zambia, all bags are off loaded onto carts and taken to the main terminal just like any other destination. Once we clear customs and pay our visa entrance fee, there is an even smaller room that receives our duffels along with every other international and national item coming into the country.

Travelers grab their bags, walk through the open doorway, and out into the parking lot to their waiting vehicles then leave. This is not the case for our team. Customs officers are waiting at the wooden counters to examine every bag tagged with our red medical label designation. Each one opened and every bottle of medication, medical supply - right down to wooden tongue blades - are examined for content, expiration dates, and packaging.

Dr. Henry and I stand ready to answer any questions, and at the same time usher our other teammates to take their personal carry-on bags and non-medical duffels out to our waiting bus. Any and all guards I have hired remain outside and are not allowed to assist us in this process.

Our team arrived in the country, and as required by the government, the nurses had to get on a small plane, after the lengthy flight with little to no sleep, and travel to the capital where we could find lodging. In the morning we would travel to the Nursing Council of Zambia located in a remote building within the city of Lusaka to seek nursing licensure.

Our arrival was prompt at 8:50 a.m. and our driver and nursing team wearing our team uniform of a colorful tropical shirt embroidered with Zambia, Africa under the OMNI logo. Our skirts, which laid no higher than our mid-calf in respect for the culture here and our documents in triplicate were notarized and in our files.

We got out of the vehicle and walked on the unleveled gravel driveway to the nursing office. Marcia, our lead nurse for the pharmacy, was to my right and twisted her ankle in a pothole. She fell hard and rolled to the ground as we all scrambled to help her. Her hand was bleeding and she complained of pain in her hand as soon as she got up. By the look of her twisted fingers, we knew it was broken.

Gil, who wasn't far behind, had bandages in her bag. We both helped Marcia to a nearby bench before we went in. We bandaged her hand, cleaned up the blood as best as we could with no water and went into the office, determined to become licensed once again.

We sat in a narrow hallway as office staff busied themselves all around us. Marcia kept her hand bandaged and elevated to keep the swelling from increasing. A woman with a tray of tea, cups, and biscuits passed by and asked if we were alright.

"Yes, we are fine," I answered for us. "Just a minor scrape on our way in." Marcia tried lifting her arm to show her.

The three of us passed the interview and were licensed once again. We returned to our waiting driver and headed to the airport for yet another flight back to Ndola so that we could meet our team. We were exhausted and ready to finally reunite with our team and get to work. Marcia's hand swelled and turned blue and green during the flight.

As our challenging situation continued, we attempted to meet up with the rest of the team, but needed fuel as soon as we arrived in Ndola. It seemed like a reasonably easy plan until we attempted to start the car after we fueled up. We were using a car that had been in storage since our last trip and the battery was dead. This seems to be a common situation in the country, and asking another traveler next to you to use jumper cables to recharge the battery, was somewhat normal.

The first man who pulled into the station appeared to have a functioning car, and was affluent in his ability to purchase fuel, understand well our needs, and agreed to the attachment of jumper cables. The charge seemed to work, we thanked him, and he drove off. We did not. The car died again. Multiple attempts to revive the vehicle did not work. All we could do was wait for another car and ask for another charge.

Within a few minutes another car pulled in; the driver looked pleasant and agreed to help us.

At this point, Dr. Henry got out of our car, and as our medical director, took his leadership role and offered his help before we started our engine.

"I don't think that you have it connected correctly," he said. And with that he switched the black and red cables to create a new connection.

Elijah started our car, and the connection not only blew out our battery, but blew out the generous man's battery as well. At the same time, the man that had helped us earlier, came walking up to us from the road and said, "My car was fine until I gave you a jump. It died just after I left the station."

Fortunately for us, all people involved were kind and gracious. Dr. Henry offered to pay for new batteries all around. The sun was setting. We had been traveling for a long time. We had no idea where our team was and worried about how to back. Then I looked across the street and saw the infamous sign: FATMOLS Lodge. It was to be our home for the next two weeks, and it was where our team had been waiting for us all day.

Our team was great; they secured the lodging rooms, moved beds, tables, and unloaded duffels. Medications only available for purchase were procured from the local pharmacy then loaded onto our bus for the clinic in the morning.

We stayed in an old musty lodge, which easily accommodated a team of eighteen. There was only one towel per room despite three or more people were in each room. Some rooms had no water and some had no electricity. It was what we expected.

That night hotel staff shut off the water and electricity. I felt desperate after so many days of travel to have water in the morning to wash up. I woke around 1 a.m. Heavy rain slapped across the windows. I got up and stepped outside our door and placed plastic bags under the rain spouts to gather water for the morning. It took longer and was harder than expected. I was exhausted, but was determined to make this work. With a full staff, a lot of water was needed.

We placed the plastic bags in the shower, on the sink, and around the floor to store until morning. I woke at sunrise. Unfortunately, all the bags leaked and there was no water left. To further discourage my futile efforts, large bugs found their way on and inside the bags. No water, no towels, and no electricity. My frustration took over and I took out my pocket knife and divided the one towel we had into four parts. I took the shredded part of the towel to each of my roommates and to my head nurse of pharmacy across the grassy lawn. We washed up that morning with bottled water and a piece of a towel.

Breakfast was meager - one small toaster and bread for the entire team. Somewhere in the lodge, the staff heated water for our tea, which they brought to our area in small amounts. We were tired, hungry, and lacking amenities for a decent start of any day ... but we had to leave. People who had nothing and who were worse off than we were this bright sunny morning were waiting us to provide health care. I climbed onto the bus with the rest of our eighteen-member team ready to serve over 600 people. We headed to our first tribal village roughly forty-five minutes away.

As our bus meandered through the bush and tall pines, it reminded me of Michigan - all the thick dense greenery. A while later, we finally came to a rock laden path that became quite treacherous for the bus especially one pulling an open trailer. There were small foot paths stretching through the bush, but no signs of people. Our driver told us that, on occasion, families of monkeys would scurry through the trails to avoid villagers.

We left the dense opening of trees, and turned right onto a more challenging dirt path full of rocks and potholes. The next left took us down to the river where tall grass and reeds grew along the banks. I was surprised to see the driver head toward a tiny wooden rickety bridge intended as a foot path to cross the flowing water. I grabbed onto the sides of the bus and prayed it would hold up as the bus, trailer, and our team drove over.

Paul, our driver, drove slowly across the weathered boards. The creaks and groans of the wood caused goosebumps to pop up all over my body. I heard everyone hold their breath as we passed over the water, and onto the other side. We were fortunate, but remembered that we had to pass this way again later in the night.

Once across the bridge, we came to the village of Mansansa. The bar made of thin wood and painted blue stood to our left. Patrons were already present and partaking in the brew. To our right sat a tiny store about six feet by eight. Sugar enhanced water in plastic bags hung from branches for people to purchase. A few eggs piled up like a pyramid were on the small wooden shelf. One bar of soap lay on the back shelf, weathered and brown, as no one could afford to purchase it. Cooking oil, in already used plastic water bottles, lined the left shelf. Business here was marginal, however, the owner had a commodity with no competition. Children with no shoes and shirts watched as we drove by - some running as they saw our white faces.

Dust blew in off the plains into our windowless structure. The cold wind blew hard causing grit to fly into our eyes, mouth, and clothing. I could not imagine how it was for the villagers who endured this every day with no clothing to insulate the elements.

The team set up the wound care station on a dirt floor in the abandoned building. Throughout the day, we were challenged with severe cases of wounds that penetrated to the bone. Gil worked her best to care for and dress these life threatening wounds. People arrived with gaping holes in their skin and cuts left unwashed due to a lack of soap. Muscles were exposed leaving the perfect entry for bacteria and further contamination. Once healthy bones were infected, requiring potent antibiotics and in some cases amputation. Patients arrived looking as though they had come from a war zone. We tended to their needs allowing them to then leave cleansed, debrided, treated, bandaged, and supplied with further items to extend their care at home.

The pharmacy suspended over 1,500 prescriptions, vitamins, birthing kits, and lifesaving antibiotics. One mother brought her mentally challenged teenage daughter to the pharmacy line for her medications. I noted a string tied around her neck with a ball of prickly thorns hanging from it at the chest area. Scarring had already occurred on her skin from months or perhaps years of wear and abrasion to that area. When I asked the mother to tell me about the brown ball of thorns around her daughter's neck she said, "My daughter is not right in her head and has fits. I took her to the witch doctor and they tried to command the demons from her. They gave us this to protect and ward off any evil spirits that are with her."

After an examination, we learned that she had pneumonia. Our instructions for the medications were clear and knew that her illness would be cured if her mother followed our directions and took the medication as prescribed. Her fits and mental status would remain the same. God bless her.

The next day we traveled to Baluba, the home to Congolese refugees and their families. Others outside the area came to this little village with the hopes of finding a place to live with little or no means. The Congo was within visual distance from our site.

Cardiac disease rarely affects a healthy woman in her twenties. Working as a triage nurse, I had to rule it out before I could dismiss the symptoms to any other source.

By late afternoon we had already treated around 400 patients with another 200 plus left to see before the sun went down. My station was triage located in the back end of the building near the pharmacy. My view consisted of patients, and graffiti on the gray cold and uneven cement block walls with no windows.

My next patient was a young woman accompanied by six children, one of them carrying a baby in her arms. Her eyes cast downward and her shoulders hung - clearly lacking confidence. She kept quiet and stood off to the side, hiding behind the others.

Through the interpreter we learned she had chest pain. My gut told me there was something else going on. I looked closer to see if there were other symptoms that could help me to determine what was going on with her. Darkness surrounded her eyes and cheeks like a mask. Her face, now red, appeared to be similar to that of a severe sunburn. Again, this did not make sense as African skin, with its dark pigmentation, protects them from the damaging rays of the sun. Her presentation did not match her complaint.

My first thought went to her husband. Women being abused by their husbands has been a common phenomenon going on throughout Africa here recently. These men not only abuse them physically, they also abuse them mentally by telling them repeatedly that they are worthless, unattractive, and have no means of being of value to their husband. This abuse creates a lack in self-confidence and pride of being a woman of color so they resort to applying bleach to their skin so they can look more like a Caucasian woman. The cream robs them of their natural beautiful deep brown skin and leaves them with scarring and signs of a chemical burn. It also robs their wallet of funds that are desperately needed for food. The source can usually be traced to a man in their life that is not happy with whom they are, or happy with himself.

My triage questions continued as one would do in a medical setting. How long have you had this pain? How severe is it? Is it constant or intermittent? When do you get this pain?

"I get the pain every two weeks when my husband gets paid," she said. Her eyes now lowering even further to avoid mine.

"What happens when he gets paid?" I asked, already suspecting the answer. I tried to make my voice as comforting as possible so that she would feel safe in answering my question.

"He gets drunk and … and he beats me." Her voice quickly weakened and went to a whisper.

I took the stethoscope from around my neck and the cuff from the table in front of me to continue her physical exam. I kept my eyes on her face, and she kept her eyes down toward her lap. The children were quiet and huddled around her like little chicks.

As I pushed up her sleeve to take her blood pressure, I saw layers of bruises and welts on her arm. Some appeared to be recent and others were starting to fade from earlier attacks.

The higher I raised the sleeve, the lower her eyes sunk to the ground. She was an abused woman no doubt. My mind raced as to how I could help her here in this country.

My first instinct was to tell her to run. Get out. Leave. Because he will eventually kill you. I couldn't help but feel empathy for her. She was a sad, lonely, fearful and controlled, mother of six. She was like a song bird in a cage hoping to be freed and not harmed while escaping.

"He is going to kill you if you don't leave," I said.

The pain in her chest was on her left rib cage caused by a punch of his fist. The pain from a fractured rib could last months and would hurt no matter what position you were in and breathing became a cruel chore.

"Why is your skin peeling and red? What are you putting on your face to make this chemical burn?" I asked.

"I want to look prettier for my husband, because he does not like me the way that I am." Her answer made my stomach hurt.

She didn't realize, and may never realize, that no matter what she does or says, he won't ever see her differently. The damage has been done. It was impossible. He abused his wife and would rather beat her, and would eventually kill her than face his own inadequacies.

"You have been born as a beautiful African woman," I said. "Born in the very image of what God wanted you to look like. Your skin, face, and soul have been made exactly how God wants you to be. Be proud of your skin, and your African heritage," I added. "I think you are beautiful just as you are." I smiled warmly. "The lotion will harm your skin and destroy the very beauty that you possess."

"If you want to leave him, and be free from this abuse, I will help you," I assured her.

I could not believe the words coming from my mouth, as I would usually have a plan in place before saying that out loud. But the words came out freely and with conviction.

She lifted her eyes for the first time and listened.

"Here is my cell phone number. If you want help, call me. I will come and get you and your children and take you away from this abuse. I will offer you a job and your children can attend the OMNI School. Please consider it." I left her with this promise.

She left; her six children following behind like a brood of baby yellow chicks. They were going where she would go and needed the comfort of her body and presence of her strength no matter how limited that could be. She walked off and I assumed that I would never see her again.

As the sun set, the compound turned into a chaotic, frenzy of people, desperate to have their needs filled before the team departed. The armed guards held back the crowd from encroaching upon the pharmacy table.

Our clinic at Baluba finished as it always does in the dark of night. Our team used head lamps to complete the prescriptions that would save lives of the more than 100 people standing in line at the pharmacy. Lights danced across the pharmacy table in hopes of keeping a visual on the medications and the prescriptions. Creativity continued as we hung a small pocket flash light from a rope suspended from a beam on the ceiling to create some form of controlled lighting over the table. We will finish the day - God willing. We are willing as well.

The team scrambled to methodically put away every last medication from the tables, load the duffels, and rush to the waiting bus with the blaze of the bonfire burning the garbage, dirty needles and used bandages as our backdrop.

I counted the heads on the bus, did a roll call, gathered the guards, and then finally Paul, our driver, ushered me onto the bus. There were still people just hanging around; children ran behind the bus wanting more. We cared for each and every one of them to the best of our abilities with what we were able to care for them with - some went home and some didn't survive. We cared for each one as though they were the only one. I always want to do more. There's never enough time. It is 8 p.m. and we haven't returned to the base all day, not eaten since 6 a.m., and needed to repeat this all over again tomorrow.

The next morning my cell phone starting ringing as our team was gathering for breakfast. *Little early*, I thought, having no idea who it could be, as the number was not in my contact list. The language and request was beyond my interpretation, so I handed my phone to Derrick, my guard who was preparing our car for the day's journey.

"It is Jane," he said over his shoulder. He continued the conversation with her in Bemba, and from what I could tell, he was trying to understand where she was. She wanted to be helped.

Apparently she waited at the highway just walking distance from her dirt house with her baby secured on her back. She was willing to leave and be free from the abuse that caged her like a tormented animal. I immediately thought of the bravery that it took to walk out that door, not look back and go for the freedom she might find. She had made a plan and with just one person agreeing to help her, she left.

The team left on the bus to the next clinic while we drove to Baluba where we found Jane in a traditional tribal cloth modest dress with the baby wrapped and balanced on her back. We slowed, motioning for her to quickly get into the back seat.

It was an unusual day. Elijah was back at the lodge and sick, so I had his car to drive. Once Jane was in the car, Derrick quickly asked her other children were and where her husband was. She indicated that she had instructed the remaining children to stay at home and not to leave until she returned with help. She also told them that if their father came by to find her, they were to tell him that she had gone to run an errand in the village.

Because we were now out of Derrick's jurisdiction of the police station, we had to go to the Baluba police and get an armed guard to accompany us to pick up the children and to register a complaint against her husband for physical abuse. We drove a few miles down the road and picked up a guard from the police post in full uniform, sporting his AK47. He got in the back and sat next to Jane, and Derrick quickly debriefed him as to the nature of our business. I was introduced as the president of OMNI and was told that a history of abuse had been revealed to me in yesterday's medical clinic.

The pace turned up a notch at that point. The police asked Jane is she was willing to file a report against her husband which would then initiate an arrest.

She was willing.

The police instructed me to go back to the police station where we could pick up another guard so that they would have two local police and Derrick to make the arrest. Back we went and picked up guard number two, also armed.

I'm back in that movie again, I thought...*and this time I'm the driver.*

Jane had told the officers that her husband volunteered at a local community clinic where he was known to steal drugs and sell them on the streets for money.

What a guy - he beats his wife and steals.

We drove in the field between banana trees until we came to a white building where a few people waited to be seen. Guard number two went inside to inquire about Jane's husband. While he was in there, I turned the car around thinking it was a good idea to be heading toward the exit for a quick getaway should things turn ugly.

To our surprise, the guard came out quickly and told us that Jane's husband had just left, to go and find Jane to kill her. He had learned from a neighbor that she had left him and suspected that she had help.

We drove back into the compound and, after a few turns on the uneven, dirt road, spotted Jane's husband on a bike. His rapid peddling and wrinkled forehead, caused by his dropped eyebrows, spoke volumes - anger. He was on the hunt.

"Stop the car," said the officer in the back.

I did and all three jumped out. They gathered around his front and sides and pulled him to the ground. As one told him he was under arrest, another handcuffed him. Once learning why he was being arrested, he immediately started arguing and denying.

The third guard opened the back hatch of the truck and helped him in. I'll never forget the angry chilling face I saw in the rear view mirror. I had to think that the car was getting a little full at this point. We had three armed guards, a woman and a baby, a prisoner, and me.

She was the mother of his six children. He was her husband, abuser, and user. His thin facade, that had fooled the public into thinking he was a family man, was over. He was a shell of a man, hollow in character but full of himself. He tried to manipulate the officer with his charm, choosing to tell lies about his recent whereabouts, and his involvement in additional activities that benefited his weak soul.

We later learned that he had a girlfriend who he had hold onto his kwatcha, the local currency that usually filled his pockets.

Jane's pockets were empty, and her children's stomachs rumbled with hunger.

I found it hard at times to remember to stay on the left side of the road. I gripped the steering wheel reminding myself that lives were depending on me - Jane, her children, and the tiny baby on her back. We had to get to the jail.

The outline of the AK47 in the rear view mirror, being held firmly by the police officer, kept grabbing my attention. The same image was to my right in the front seat.

The already overloaded car was about to get more crowded as we now had to go to Jane's house a few blocks away and pick up her five children and any personal possessions that she wanted. The children, dressed in torn and dirty clothes, were waiting patiently for their mother's return. Each one stood in the front barren yard. Nothing seemed to flourish there - no grass or vegetation of any kind, and especially not small children and their mother.

We pulled up in front of the dreary shambles of a building that she called home. Almost a perfect square made of block cement, probably by hand, the walls of the house were not straight and parts of the wall was crumbling. The roof was various lengths of tin and were held down at the seams with large rocks. No glass was to be found in the few openings that served as windows. A ragged piece of cloth hung over the door frame to serve as a division from the outside to the dismal inside.

A worn down red dirt path led straight to the front door from off into the fields somewhere in the distance - a path well-traveled. My heart fluttered the moment I spotted a board game, complete with small stones nestled in tiny cup marks, carved into the hard ground. Tiny fingers had sculpted the earthen board creating hours of entertainment out of nothing. Two of Jane's children were sitting on the ground playing the game in the dirt.

Jane led us into the house. All but two of the guards stayed near our vehicle to secure and keep vigil of the cuffed prisoner in the back. Our eyes had to adjust from the bright sun outside to the damp darkness that filled the house. The hole in the roof that was over the hallway had been patched at some point by a section of tin to hold out the rain. The tin appeared to be the only value in the house.

The man had provided next to nothing for his wife and six children. A mid-sized dented pot served as the kitchen. An empty corn sack and a handmade broom made of elephant grass bound by a rubber strip similar to a black rubber band was the only cleaning item I saw. There was no sign of any food.

A dirt-packed path led us to a small bedroom in the back where two dirty blankets heaped in the corner functioned as the bed for the five children. No clothes or toys could be seen.

Across the narrow galley of the hall was the bedroom that Jane and her husband occupied. A dirty worn mattress void of bedding was pushed up against the dirt wall.

There was nothing to gather in any of these rooms, except bad memories. We walked the short distance to the living room where there was an old torn sofa chair and a small, low wooden table. One had to assume that this chair was for the husband, who arrogantly ruled the house. Jane's eyes quickly scanned the room as she walked over to a box on a shelf that contained a mess of papers and documents. She rifled through them until she found what she wanted. In the group of papers were the identification papers and national cards for her children and herself. Included in the lot that she needed was the immunization cards that the government provided when her children received their free immunizations as infants.

Beyond the papers, was a plastic bag filled with clothing that appeared to be hers and that of her children. She grabbed the bag, put the papers in her blouse and indicated that she was ready to leave. There wasn't much, but at least she had documentation for her and her children.

She was making a courageous move for her and her family. She moved in a determined fashion as she had protection now from the monster that was being held in the car. The guard carried the bag for her and we exited out into the sunshine toward the car - careful to step over the board game carved in the earth. No one looked back as they piled back into the back seat of our SUV.

I was driving and had no idea where we would go next. Derrick was in the front seat on my right and was clearly in his element to complete this arrest and to find a safe place for this family. I felt as though I was in a movie. I had conviction, however, to make a safe place for this abused women and her children.

I looked back into the second seat of the over packed vehicle to see Jane, the baby on her back, and five small children huddled around her like baby chicks under a hen. In the far back sat the man who now, finally had no control over them and was rendered harmless at least for the moment. He glared at Jane and then at me.

I turned to Jane and said, "I don't want you to turn around and make eye contact with him, as he is trying to intimidate you and me, but it is not going to work. You are safe now and he can't get to you anymore. He won't get to me either." I was grateful for his handcuffs and for the armed men who backed me up.

Jane started to look back out of habit and fear.

"Jane, you need to keep looking forward. Don't let him get to you," I pleaded. I kept an eye on the prisoner, and one on the road.

He kept making verbal gestures to Jane, which was quickly halted by the verbal order coming from the guard. This was going to be a long drive into town, and I knew we had to get to the jail as soon as we could. We had about forty miles to go.

Before we could leave Baluba jurisdiction, we had to drop off the two guards as they could not leave their area of command. Derrick suggested that we drive the guards to their police station where Jane could make a formal complaint against him and there, he would be imprisoned. From there we had about a thirty-minute ride to reach our destination.

As I took in the events that had happened already by mid-morning, I knew that my team was back at another clinic site and that I needed to get back to help. We had no contact with them and knew that they had no idea of what we were doing. It was a tenuous situation. I was also driving someone else's car and had no written permission or verification that I should be at the steering wheel, or in this position. This is how it goes here, and we were already deep into this scenario.

I decided to pick up speed so that we could get to the jail sooner. As we came up over a slight hill, there on the side of the road was something that I have never seen in the thirteen years of working here in Zambia. It was new, out of place and totally unexpected, and it had blue lights flashing from its roof. This was totally out of character and certainly was foreign to this area.

In a matter of minutes, I was being pulled over by one of the only three new police cars in the entire country. I pulled over and came to a quick halt at the side of the road. I kept my hands on the steering wheel.

"You do have your international license don't you, Karen?" Derrick asked. He leaned forward to see what my response would be and at the same time to acknowledge the large uniformed man that was leaving his vehicle and rapidly approaching my side of the car.

"Well I have a license ... but..." I knew what he meant as I hesitated.

"Let me take care of this and just do as I say," he said calmly as the patrol officer approached our vehicle and asked for my license. Derrick pulled out his ID badge and his officer license. "Detective Sergeant Kalinda here," he said calmly and with authority.

It was apparent that they knew each other and had some history of other work related encounters. I felt grateful for that. "We are taking a prisoner to the jail in Twapia," Derrick said as he pointed to Jane's husband in the far rear of our vehicle.

As the officer peered further into our car, leaning against my shoulder, looking past Jane, her six children and far into the very back for a better view, to see Jane's husband raising his cuffed hands as though to prove our declaration of his presence.

266

There was a short pause as the officer pulled his body back from the window where I was sitting, holding my breath, and remaining looking forward. Derrick sat next to me and appeared confident for both of us.

"Ok, Ok, Sergeant, you can go on ahead. I was going to stop you, for speeding but I can see that you are on official business," he stated in a firm tone. He looked at me a second time and am sure that he had questions, but refrained from asking. I sat there with both hands firmly on the steering wheel and looked forward hoping not to make eye contact.

"Thank you, sir, and have a good day," Derrick said.

"Yes, thank you," I replied.

"You are most welcome, Madam. Next time we will discuss your license," he said almost in a whisper.

It never came up again.

I smiled and drove on with just a slight ease off the gas pedal. He was my protector, and protector of many. *Priceless,* was all that came to mind.

I released a heavy sigh of relief as we drove off toward Twapia.

I had been to the Twapia Jail before on business with other infractions against patients and knew the way. We turned right off the main road, went a couple kilometers and turned left. The jail was on our left and was always open for business.

We arrived at the small jail, a building painted teal with a white stripe of paint in the middle running horizontal and parallel to the ground. Derrick escorted Jane's husband into the small office that was used as an intake room. I followed behind cautiously.

Once inside the office, a young woman officer in uniform approached him and told him empty his pockets of all items. A bundle of kwatcha, the country's currency, was found crumpled up in both pockets - $40 - more than most people here make in a month.

It is more than likely that this money was profit that he had received from the stolen medications at the clinic where he worked. Ironically, he had told Jane that he had no money to buy them food that week. *How can one man be such a disgrace*, I thought. How can this man have no character other than his own selfish needs?

He was placed in the corner on the floor and told to sit there while the paperwork was filed.

Despite his lowly position on the floor, an arrogant attitude of entitlement remained on his face. This man would not likely change by this incarceration.

Jane agreed to file a formal complaint against him for physical abuse; a charge that would have him imprisoned. Her bruises and welts were clearly seen by the officer. According to the law of Zambia, a written statement from a physician who has examined the victim must also accompany the complaint. X-rays would need to be taken as well to determine if any bones were broken or ribs cracked. I could see clearly that our next stop was going to be Ndola General Hospital.

Hospitals are prepared for abuse cases and interestingly enough, so are those in a third world country in Africa. It was surprising to me to see how Jane was ushered in before other people who were waiting to be seen by a doctor. Her case was marked as a criminal investigation. Our guard, complete with his gun, and my presence in a white team shirt, AKA a woman from America bringing in a woman from Africa to be evaluated, may have moved us to the front of the long line when we arrived. I don't know, but what I do know is that physical abuse is not tolerated and is prosecuted by the law.

Her chest x-rays showed multiple rib fractures in various stages of healing. Friday of June, Friday of May, Friday night of April. Everything was recorded in black and white on the shadows of the x-ray and were documented on the intake form for domestic violence cases. We had the evidence that we needed along with her testimony. We thanked the doctors and paid the $12 due for exams and x-ray fees. This whole process for us was procedural. For Jane, this was a breakthrough and was her pathway to be free from abuse once and forever. She remained polite, soft in her demeanor, and glanced at me from time to time with appreciation.

We headed back to the jail in Twapia where her husband was now escorted and placed behind bars - cement block cells with iron bars open to the air. I could hear the large metal key secure the lock and the

269

door slam shut. In the corner of the room a cement ledge served as a bed with no bedding. Food would not be provided either, as these luxuries need to come from the family members. In this case, the family member was not willing to supply these comforts. We suspected his night was going to be a long one. Pity was in short supply that day as we walked away from the cold iron bars that retained him.

In all of these travels, we had six children in the car, one of them being a small baby of whom I held during the x-rays. Their sad faces held back emotions that they could not understand. I had given out all of my granola bars, candy, gum, and water to them throughout the day - there was nothing was left to give. I knew that they were getting hungry and night was coming. We headed back to the OMNI site where promises of a home, a job, and an education for the children were present.

Once inside our secured gates, I took Jane to the interior of our administration building at the school which would be transformed into her new temporary home. This building was originally built a few years ago as a school building with four classrooms, a main gathering room, a kitchen, and a bathing room with two showers and three toilets. There was electricity, running water, and security, all of which Jane never had.

In the storage room, were six iron beds and mattresses stacked to the ceiling. Dishes, bedding, blankets, and some clothing were still there from the overseas container that had been shipped by us the year before and not yet utilized. Someone back in the states had donated these items in hopes of helping someone.

They did and it was perfect.

We went through the boxes, duffle bags, and dusty boxes that had sat in this room for a couple of years waiting for the right family in need. That family was here and we were all thrilled. It was like Christmas for them and it showed on their faces.

We had pillows and a few outdated curtains that worked perfectly for Jane and her family. The building came together flawlessly. I couldn't get this amazing experience out of my head. I did, however, feel bad about leaving the team and the patients behind at today's clinic.

I was meant to be here - I had traveled to the other side of the world for this moment and for this family, it was worth every minute, every dollar, and every effort - priceless at every turn.

The guards and I moved beds, pulled down boxes, and started to transform the administration building into the most beautiful home these children and mother had ever seen. I found sheets and made them into curtains, nailing them to the wall and using duct tape where necessary. It was a miracle - we had everything we needed for this family, including the right size clothing. The children had beds with colorful sheets and blankets for the first time in their lives.

I had the guard go into the village and buy a bag of meal, cooking oil, and kapenta. We had a tray of eggs in the kitchen, left from this week's layers, within walking distance on the property. Dinner would be greater than they had had in a long time. Safety was a gift that perhaps they had never had. What else could we hope for besides full stomachs, clean beds, and security. The day was more than successful and rewarding beyond description.

Jane started cleaning the kitchen and the children were excited to be in a building with lights, space to run around, food, and most of all, safety. Jane had a home here within the gates of OMNI. Here her children were safe and the abuser was behind bars. The youngest child, that could walk, was only three and clung to me as we went through the building creating a home. She had been the fallout child - left to fend for herself while her mother tended to the baby and fended off her abusive father. I picked her up and kept her with me as we went about the building. She hung on like a Velcro child, and seemed content. So was I. We had saved a woman and her six children. Thanks be to God.

I think of Jane so very often and have learned a great deal about myself from her. She was courageous, not knowing what the future would hold, but stepped out in faith, leaving the neglect and punishment behind, taking children with her, and facing the world on her own. Life for her without abuse ... without control ... was worth taking the risk to move ahead to a life that is new and safe.

Be free Jane and flourish!

When I arrived back in the U.S. from the medical mission, the house remained empty, a small sticky note remained on the counter, and he was gone. I filed for divorce the next day. I was sad that thirty-six years of marriage was over.

I have come to realize that we are not born with courage but it is something that we have to develop. With each step toward courage there is an element of fear. I had to have the courage to leave the life that I once thought that we had, and accept the life that is now given to me. Once the fear is overcome the courage is strengthened. Without taking the risk to develop courage we lose out in life and fear remains. Jane left the abuse and her abuser making the only positive step forward to make life better.

Jane and I have few words when we see each other, but we know that life is better indeed and we smile and hug each other as song birds who have survived outside of the cage.

Jane has worked with OMNI for the past three years as a domestic caretaker at the OMNI School. Her raw reddened cheeks have healed and her ebony glow had returned. Gloria, her oldest daughter, graduated from the seventh grade and, with a sponsor, has continued on to the eighth grade in a government school nearby. She now rents her own small home and can provide for her family on the income that OMNI pays her each month. She is a survivor and her courage and strength is admirable. There is a saying in Africa that rain beats the hide of a leopard, but it cannot wash away its spots. I think that is true of Jane as well. She is a survivor.

As rewarding as it is to save a woman from her abuser, it is equally as frustrating and devastating to not be able to produce those same results when facing other obvious crimes against humanity.

Mansansa is home to rural substance farmers who are barely capable of surviving off the land and where hunger is known by many. In this small town it is rare for anyone to afford an education, health care, or any amenities in life. The bare necessities of food and shelter are beyond the reach of each family. OMNI ventures into this vast remote tribal region every year and provides health care to the masses, usually over 600 needy individuals in one day.

It's a tough location despite the beautiful drive through the tall trees deep in the hills of Zambia, closer to the Congo border than our clinic had been before. This time, our team set up the clinic in an abandoned split wood building, with no windows, no electricity, no doors, but had a breathtaking view of the tropical palms that line the river bed that flows through the village. The people gather in front of the building with hope that OMNI will take care of them.

And, we do.

Silvia, a thirteen-year-old child born into a family of twelve - ten children - in the village of Mansansa, is just one of the many families.

Food, as was for many, came sparingly for Silvia's family as did compassion. Silvia was sold to an older man in the village in exchange for food for the rest of the family from time to time. She became his child bride the same year. She came to us pregnant at age fourteen and did not know when her baby was due, or the full name of her husband. She knew that he worked somewhere, but was unsure of the location or what he did to make money - she was a classic case with the same demeanor as the other girls and women who had been beaten, but would not divulge their abuser.

Her mother, the saleswoman in this human transaction, accompanied her to the clinic and offered little as far as medical history or social background, clearly hiding her transgressions.

I took the young girl into the makeshift exam room and tried to find a heartbeat with the fetal doppler. We had no exam table and no lights, so we placed a surgical drape on the cold dirt floor and asked her to lie down, supporting her head with a towel from the duffel. As luck would have it, or in this case - not, the Doppler failed to work that day.

Upon exam, I could feel that the baby's head was down, and that she appeared, according to the height of the fundus, to be about seven months pregnant. Silvia, could not tell me if the baby had moved and clearly had a learning disability that prevented her from understanding her current situation. I placed my hands on either side of her abdomen and moved the baby from side to side gently, until I got a response of motion. It was the best that I could get at the time as she laid on a thin tarp on the dirt floor of our building. Light shined in through the window that had no pane, and dirt blew in as the strong winds of winter pushed against the building outside. It was cold and damp in there, but we had a live fetus, and that made me happy.

We helped her up and took her back to the triage station where I asked her more questions - things were not adding up quite yet. After a barrage of questions, attempting to flush out the truth, the mother admitted to selling her daughter to rid her of her responsibilities for her. The husband would come home and beat his pregnant wife and then the mother. Beatings were in exchange for food, and whatever insignificant items that he may bring into their home. He was a dangerous man, and living under his abuse was even more dangerous than going without food. His presence could be lethal.

It was story like the rest, another crime against humanity. Our senior guard took a statement from the mother of Silvia. She was then arrested and put in jail for selling her daughter. A warrant was issued for the husband, who remained at large when we left.

Knowing the determination of the police to protect Silvia and to remove her perpetrator, I prayed that his arrest would be before the sun came up the next morning. A baby however, was soon to be born to a child who was unprepared to provide the necessary care to survive. Strong winds blew, laden with dust and dirt, as we left the village, and tomorrow would bring another day in Mansansa. Mother Zambia, fair and beautiful woman, tend to, heal, and care for your babies, for they are your future.

The Village of George: Put Dirt on My Grave

The British left in 1964, and Zambia gained its independence. Little remained unchanged for years, except the knowledge that everything must be done by "the book." In many rural areas, there was no electricity, no clean potable water, no infrastructure, and no plumbing except outdoor holes dug into the ground surrounded if you were fortunate by a three-sided woven mat wall. Substance farming is the main source of survival, and even that does not meet the needs of every family. The margins are very tight, and most people go to bed hungry at night with no means of providing a meal for the following day. Bare feet, and torn clothes adorn the small children who run among the few goats and free range chickens.

Industry and commerce does not exist anywhere in the village of thatched huts and mud shanties. The wealthiest man in the village owns the local pub where home brew is served out of sixty-gallon oil drums open to the air. Mice have dangerously tried to navigate the rim of the drums often fall into the brew to their death. The owner scoops them out and throws them in the nearby garbage pile, leaving traces of their remains at the bottom of the brew, unseen by those who indulge in this toxic solution.

Small rocks piled one on top of each other in a staggering tower, knee level marking the paths that lead to the handmade containers indicating that the brew is done.

Life in this village can be tough. We had walked out of the village the year before and watched as a mother hen and her chicks were moving through the dirt relocating to a safer place. Out from the end row of maize came a cobra, poised in an upward and erect position, and struck with lightening force at a chick, rendering it lifeless. The children screamed, picked up rocks and, with their little bare feet, ran toward the snake chasing it back into the rows of corn.

A few minutes later they returned with the dead cobra draped over a long stick. Cheers came from the children that did not accompany the brave group into the field and together they placed their day's hunt in a tree - hanging for all villagers to see. Triumph over evil, gentleness over force, life over death ... justice served.

It's also a peaceful place except for occasional domestic violence justified by the man's lack of intolerance to women during his drunken stupors. Death is common here as there is no health care, no education, and no access to government assistance. Mid-life is around sixteen years and people rarely live to see old age. Time is measured by events and not hours in the day or years. Few know what year they were born, and many have no birth certificate indicating their existence.

This is where OMNI's home base is, among the poorest of the impoverished. It is a farming community walking distance to the southern border of the hills of the Congo. Most people here have never been into the nearest city as it is too far to walk and no one has money once they get there.

Our mobile clinic set up under the large shade trees inside what George claimed as their city center. The robin's egg blue painted cement building topped with a thin tin roof and cement floors was the meeting hall for the entire village. The brilliant blue paint was chipped and created a beautiful backdrop for the dark brown skinned children that ran past its walls. Inside were three rooms with similar chipped paint, no electricity and wooden doors that had been handmade, and never leveled to match the door frame.

Over 500 people lined up to access health care for the first time in their lives. Women with babies, women who were pregnant with babies on their backs, orphans with grandparents, and a hand full of elderly made their way to our clinic.

As the day progressed, a thin man appeared through the crowd pushing an old bicycle carrying a slumped over elderly man on the back fender. He was supported in a nearly upright position and a completing his journey to us. I left my post and walked over to him and together lowered the man to the ground where he lay almost motionless. The bike had no kickstand, as it had probably broken off years ago, and was leaned against the tree. It was the ambulance for the village, simple, offering no siren, no flashing lights, no emergency support or means of medical intervention. It was simply a bike with two worn wheels that provided transportation for the critical patients in the village.

"How long has he been like this?" I asked the interpreter. I had not learned enough yet to be able to communicate without his help.

"He fell ill two days ago, has not eaten or drank since then. He lives alone, except for his seven-year-old grandson," the interpreter said.

I knelt on the hard ground next to him and could see his eyes glazed and showing signs of his deteriorating condition. Jaundice had set in, his pulse was rapid and weak and his respirations were shallow and labored. He was emaciated and dehydrated, and smelled of urine to no fault of his own. I knew that he was near death and wondered how he had survived even this long alone.

"Where is the little boy, and who is caring for him?" I asked, worrying that a small child had been the only caretaker this man had and was now facing losing his grandfather.

How frightening it must be for him to see this man in this condition and not have another adult to go to.

I was told that the young boy was alone and wondered from neighbor to neighbor getting some nshima or bread where he could.

"What is his name so that I might address him please?" I asked.

"Emmanuel or "God is with us", said the interpreter. As he lay at my bent knees, he clearly and had very little time left on this earth. If we were in the States, he would be transferred to a health care facility or allowed to be in his home surrounded by loving family until his death. We had neither here, so our choices were limited.

"I want to go home to die," the man told the interpreter. I could only imagine him being alone with no one, and his grandson bearing the unspeakable burden of an adult situation with the limited skills of a child. "I want to go home....and have my funeral."

I was not sure that I understood him correctly, but I knew what he had just asked for. He wanted to have a funeral now, while he was alive, and know that there would be someone to put dirt on his grave. It was a simple last request, not to go without being granted. It was a gift that we could give, requiring nothing but compassion.

Our only vehicle was our team bus, similar to that of an old blue school bus with double bench seats and a single aisle down the middle. It was not the type of vehicle that would be conducive to carrying a dying man through the goat paths of this tiny African village, yet it would have to do.

We wrapped Emmanuel in a blue paper surgical drape that had covered one of our exam tables as he was cold and wet from being incontinent. Rick picked up his thin, frail body and I carried his dangling thin legs as we struggled up the two narrow steps of the old bus. We laid him on the aisle as the benches were too short to accommodate his long willowy body.

His clothes were filthy, and many sizes too large for his withered body. His frail frame seemed to be lost somewhere beneath the fabric that at one time fit him sufficiently. The ride to his hut was bumpy and difficult for the driver to navigate through the narrow dirt walking paths to his home. He spoke not a word, closing his eyes for his final journey home.

Unloading his near lifeless body was as cumbersome as it was to enter the bus due to the narrow passage of the double door entrance and the short cascade of stairs. Rick took great care as he cradled the man in his arms, legs dangling from his bent knees.

Emmanuel's house was a small dirt structure with a weathered thatched roof, patched with irregular pieces of hand-cut tin held down with random rocks. The front door had no handle and had a piece of dirty rope where the door knob should have been. Inside was dark despite the light of the day, and our eyes could not adjust immediately to the lack of light. An old cloth blocked one small window, and an empty tin can propped against the sill held the fabric back. I backed into a small irregular opening in the wall as I carried the lower end of his body, feeling a piece of fabric, rough like a grain bag fall over my back. It sent shivers down my spine as I didn't know what I was backing into or who or what was there in the dark.

We laid him down carefully and covered him with the old blanket, putting one of our jackets under his head. It was to be his final resting place, the very place that his soul would leave his exhausted body. We joined hands around him, praying to God for his comfort and his final departure from this earth. He was still alive, but we gave him a funeral, just what he wanted. He could hear us and was in full attendance.

Emmanuel died that night in his home after his funeral and where he needed and wanted to be. He was buried in a nearby local cemetery, and a piece of tumbleweed was placed in his front door signifying his death. We were honored to be with him and honored to perform his funeral.

His grandson stayed with the neighbors until a distant uncle from another province could travel several days later to get him.

"You were not alone Emmanuel, and you remain with us still." You made it home and there is dirt on your grave, as you wished.

The Challenge: Trust

Trust is defined as a firm belief in the confidence of honesty, integrity, reliability, and responsibility that one will do what he or she has said or implied. It is to believe that above all, you will not harm me for your personal gain. It is my most challenging struggle and one that I find myself trying to move forward with and give all involved the benefit of doubt. Without that faith, we would have, should have stopped years ago. Moving forward in faith does not mean that you won't get hurt, cheated out of, or swindled into something that does not benefit all. It does give you the strength, knowing that God is always with you to move forward and continue the work that you have been called to do.

I was in South Africa, actually in a market in Johannesburg years ago, and wanted to purchase a handmade doll, if you will, that resembled a tribal figure in that region. She was about four feet tall, dressed in tribal clothing, complete with beading, neck rings, and all of the colors that would adorn a woman if she were human. Once a price was agreed upon, and we made the deal for me to purchase her, I asked that the men and women in the market name her for me. "Give her a name that would be noble for this woman. "

"Numsa" was given from each of them. "For the good of us all." I loved the name and so hoped that it would be a blanket of grace that would precede all of my encounters in Africa.

Greed is everywhere, and even when you do all that you can to help another, and give what you can, greed seeps in and creates an infestation within a pure dream that wants to take more than one deserves or has worded for.

Lying awake at night for me is a reoccurring event. How can we move forward and help if we continue to be taken advantage of? Laborers work very little, and, when they see a small opening, run to the labor office and file a claim that they did not receive back pay, over pay, holiday pay, overtime, food allowance, housing allowance, all the while stealing from us while we are here working to make the next donation to their country. I get weary, but keep praying for strength to help those that are in need.

OMNI has had a 100% donation to the people policy. If you give a dollar to us, it all goes to the people. It does and has. What pains me is the greedy that intercept our good will and pad their own pockets. Perhaps, it is the survival of the fittest. Perhaps, it is greed amplified.

Hank, who had been receiving food on a monthly basis for years as he cared for little Anne, was a prime example of greed. He had more food than anyone in the small village, and had health care provided when our team was in town. He was eager to volunteer with the team as an interpreter but it was clear that his motives were other than genuine.

It was easy to see his self-serving maneuvers as he would steal vitamins and supplies off of the top pharmacy table when he thought no one was looking. He would then ask for supplies at the end of the day for sick neighbors, and relatives who he claimed could not make it that day. We were on to him and gave very little that was not verified as a legitimate need.

Astonishing Protector

Upon arrival, as always, and at sometimes requested, the recently hired guards for this mission would be lined up just outside of the airport Quonset for my inspection, introduction, and final approval. It was always in my curiosity to see who was hired, who was selected from the police force of the country, and who was the best to be chosen to protect our team and protect and secure my activities while in country.

We had a variety of guards - tall, short, young, interested, bored, disengaged, and energetic - to be included in our mission ... a well-rounded team. Most were dedicated to their work, strong, and very well trained. Their service of protection has always been appreciated and welcomed.

We had very few who ever made it beyond the gates of clearance from customs, my very starting gate for the endurance race to treat the impoverished. I would greet, shake hands, look them in the eye, assess, and determine within a few minutes who would protect my life for the next fourteen days, and who would protect the team as they traveled and worked in distant and remote areas.

I was particularly amused and amazed that one could report for duty in a drunken stupor, and expect to be hired and go unnoticed. They more than likely were not going to be effective even in a sober state. They were an immediate termination, without pay. No apologies, no pay and no regrets, thanks but no thanks. I had a few of them and I don't remember their names.

Who I do remember, and will always be grateful to, are two men, exceptional in their line of service, excelling in professionalism and admirable character. Their professional protection for my safety remains with me and fills me with great gratitude. They are the astonishing officers, true gentlemen that have guarded my life and provided safety.

Our plane landed on the tarmac of the capital and our team exited from the small aircraft gathering together for a quick picture before we entered the small airport tunnel to be approved by immigrations and fill out our visa entry cards. We walked without hesitation to the entrance and kept together as a group as I had advised. An armed, uniformed guard stood at attention near the perimeter of the pavement and addressed me with a question:

"Are you Ms. ReMine?" He asked.

I looked around, quickly thinking that we must have not completed our entry papers correctly, perhaps had violated some unknown law or rule, not familiar to me despite this being my 35th trip to this country. I hesitated to answer, but finally said, "Yes, and who are you, Sir?"

"I am Daniel, your personal guard. Give me your passport and come with me." Fright or flight sprang across my mind - but only for moment. I have taught my team never to part with your passport, never leave it or give it to anyone. I felt myself handing over the most important document that I have in my possession to a man that I did not know. I had nowhere to go and no other answer to give him other than, "It's a pleasure to meet you, Sir."

He ushered me into the airport, staying close and attentive. He was to be my protector and advisor for the next two weeks, in situations that I had no idea were about to unfold.

Daniel wore a uniform every day on our assignment, carrying an AK47, on some days, and some days appeared to not be armed. I learned that he always carried a weapon, but I didn't know what it was or where the weapon was kept. Our clinics were held in various tribal locations often times in rural places where there was little chance of protecting me from the 800 people that showed up for our clinics.

There were times that I knew he was watching me and those around me. There were times that I thought he wasn't watching and would make an attempt to slip away unnoticed, simply to check and see if he was attentive. It didn't work. When I turned around to see if I had managed to walk away, he was there, fifty feet behind, determined to keep me safe. Daniel was a professional, had guarded the former president of the country, and also had the same name as one of my sons. I began to trust him more than other guards I had employed in the past. He was a constant force field of protection from all angles. He was an incredible young man with a great deal of expertise and integrity and I was blessed to know him and have him on our team.

Later in the week, our team was invited to a business dinner across town in a community building. I was instructed to wait for the driver and Daniel to pick me up and have the team go ahead with the bus to arrive on time. The bus left with the entire team and all our contents, while I remained at the lodge for Daniel and the driver to arrive. Twenty minutes had passed and still no car, no driver, and no Daniel. I called to find out their location and to inquire why they were late. "Sorry, ma'am, there is traffic and we will be there in a few minutes," the driver said.

Another twenty minutes passed and again, no one arrived to take me to the event. Being late for a business event, in my books, was not acceptable. I called again to see where they were, thinking he was not as attentive as I had originally thought. "We will be right there, sorry again, ma'am," came the answer.

Within five minutes, the OMNI car pulled into the driveway. Daniel exited wearing a dark suit, no weapon visually seen and opened the back door of our vehicle giving a signal with his arm for me to get into the car. He closed the door and got into the left front of our car and locked the doors. There was no explanation of their tardy arrival.

"Why were you so late, and where have you both been? I was to be at the dinner forty-five minutes ago to greet the president of the club. I hope that you both have a good explanation for this delay."

Silence hung in the air. It did not seem like either man wanted to answer my question. Both men looked at each other and then looked forward with what seemed to be conviction in their voice. "There has been a threat against you this evening," Daniel said calmly. I would not let you go to the dinner without me checking it out completely before your arrival. I have been at the club, circled the outside of the building, and its interior and have spoken to the staff in regards to security. You will be watched, and I will provide security for you as you to go to the dinner."

I sat back slowly, realizing that going there was risky, but I had to trust the level of security that Daniel was providing. My heart pounded. I had no choice but to go and greet everyone in the facility and maintain complete composure.

"I don't know what to say other than, thank you," I said.

We traveled through the town, now covered in darkness, and I wondered what or who would be there to greet us. The threat had come from a former employee that had been terminated earlier for significant reasons of breach of trust and theft. He held a grudge that he had chosen to justifiably acted upon.

We arrived at the club and parked the car in the dark lot just outside the meeting hall. We walked together up the cement stairs where I could hear laughter and our team enjoying the evening. The room that we entered was filled with people, our team, club members, some known and most unknown to me. I walked in feeling secure that Daniel was at my side and would be there to protect me. I stepped in and greeted the president of the club, and those around him. I turned to introduce Daniel, and to my surprise, he was gone. I was alone and immediately thought that perhaps I had misinterpreted his loyalty and expertise. *Why would he not stay by me for protection especially when there had been a threat against my security and safely?*

My heart raced. I felt vulnerable now that I was alone in a room of strangers with no protection. There was no one on the team that I could inform of the current situation without alarming them, so I held the information to myself. I looked across and around the room for Daniel and he was no longer there, except to reappear from time to time from different doorways, always making eye contact if I looked up. He was doing his job, securing the perimeter of the building, watching the doors behind me and taking in every move in the room. He was protecting as he was trained. I was learning how to be protected, a concept that before this was foreign to me here in this country and at home.

During dinner, I was seated next to the president of the club and other members of both our team and the rotary. I chose a spot with an empty chair to my left. Daniel sat across from me. He did not eat, drink, or socialize. In a short time, he was up again and gone. I continued to see him across the room in various locations. Each time I looked at him, he made eye contact, and then was gone. The evening was uneventful from that point on, and my safety and that of the team was provided by Daniel.

The following day, we were making rounds on the home feeding programs that OMNI provided in the various villages. For a couple of months, we had been giving formula and baby clothes to a newborn double orphan who was being cared for by her aunt after her mother died post-delivery. The home was an orange brick structure with no running water or electricity, and just walking distance through the other houses from the dirt trail that people used.

We arrived at the home bringing powdered formula and blankets for the baby. It was my first visit, but our staff had been coming there for many weeks. The baby was tiny but thriving. The aunt seemed to be doing well with the baby and there was definitely a bond between the two of them. She held her close to her face and kissed her cheeks. She was proud to hand her over to me and allow me to hold her so that I could examine her to see what her state of health was. The baby was fairly well nourished and seemed to be alert. She had all of her fingers, toes, arms and legs, moving and thriving. I was concerned about her nutrition in the fact that her birth mother had died.

We agreed to continue to have canned powered formula delivered every month to supplement the baby's nutritional needs. Foster claimed that he delivered milk and cooking oil to the home every two weeks. I prayed that this was so.

Daniel was standing behind me as I held the orphaned baby and was actually hidden from our site. He continued to watch the various paths that lead to the home. The compound was made up of desperate people that watched my movements and pathway to reach this house.

I left after handing the tiny baby back to the aunt, thanking her for her care, and walked back down the dirt trail to our waiting vehicle. It was an uneasy feeling, but I was being cared for by my guard and was able to return to our vehicle without an incident.

We started our exit from the village down the narrow path with hut, shack, and people to our right and left.

"Stop please. I want to see this woman who is preparing her meal," I asked.

We stopped and I reached for the handle to get out but Daniel was already at my door to stop my exit.

"What do you want?" Daniel asked.

"I just want to get out and ask this woman what she is preparing and if I could purchase her wooden stick to bring back to the U.S. It would help people there to know how much is needed here for the families." Daniel stopped me there and would not let me exit the vehicle.

The woman sat in the back of her dirt house under a tin roof that was badly needed for repair. She sat on a tree stump and was using a wooden rounded stick to pound the vegetables that lay in the bottom of a wooden vessel. The vegetables would be added to the maize she had boiling inside to make nshima.

"Please offer her twenty dollars for her wooden vessel and stick. I will bring it back to use it to help bring more funds in to feed our

293

children," I stated. I felt awkward and ugly to ask to purchase her kitchen tools, but knew that it would help more than we could imagine at this moment.

Daniel walked back to her outdoor station and offered the funds to purchase her wooden kitchen tools. I could see that she worried about his approach and perhaps even thought that she may be in trouble. A conversation took place of which none of us in the car could see, but were watching as every word took place.

She got up and clapped and did several curtsies as she received the money in kwatcha. Her wooden vessel and the long stick that she used to pound the food for her meal were given to Daniel. He walked back to the car with both in his hands. The money that she received was more than her family could earn in a month.

Daniel put the wooden kitchen tool in the back of our car and got back into the front of the car and was quiet as he always was. We drove forward, and I finally had to ask him if what I did was alright.

"You blessed their family with money that they did not have. She can purchase another grinding vessel for very little. This gift will bless them for many days." He looked forward and remained stately.

I felt fortunate that Daniel was in our life. He was a fine gentleman with a deep soul rooted in doing good deeds for others. I sat in the back, and admired his solid character and his integrity. I valued the fact that he provided safety for me always. That was priceless as we saw. I don't know how to explain that further as it seems far too inadequate.

His last day with me included accompanying me and the team to the airport to see us off for our return flight to the states. It is a process leaving the country as a team. We leave what we can behind for those in need. We pack what we need to bring home, mostly dirty clothes and such into duffels that once housed medications. We also wrap items that we have purchased in those very same bags to take home to family and friends as our offering for being gone so long.

The ride to the airport for me was solemn. I miss everyone so much when I depart and really would rather stay for another month or longer. For some on our team, there may be a desire to finally go home, get back into the luxuries of our existence and be done with this experience. Some are change forever, and are not sure what going home means. Can they go home unchanged? Can they go home and explain even in the slightest way what we saw, did and took into our souls?

Nonetheless, we have to go, as our visas dictate that. We file out of the bus, into the tin covered airport of Zambia in the north and make our way back to the U.S.

We put our bags, personal packs, and items purchased requiring hand carrying on the conveyor belt that would x-ray the contents. Our phones, ID in the form of passports, all go through the conveyer belt. All bags went through and would be picked up at the other side once we cleared the scanner for our bodies. Once on the other side we gathered up our belongings and moved on to the counter for check in.

As one of our team members passed through the metal detector and into the restricted zone, the conveyor belt stopped, backed up, and was paused for further viewing and investigation.

A slight shift in the guard's position on his stool and then a motion for another customs agent to come and view the bag indicated that one of our team members was being stopped for their bag's contents. The machine had picked up the image of a large rock, picked from our site as a souvenir to take home.

"Open the bag, and let us see what you have," came the order from the agent.

Upon inspection, it was clearly a rock, of no value and of no significance, weighing about five to six pounds. "You can't take this, and I have to fine you for this," came the next piece of information. I saw it as I was watching all team members going into the line. It was audible to many in the small airport that a discussion of escalating tone was taking place.

Daniel was already inside the restricted area and was standing against the wall watching all activities of our team in a one hundred and eighty-degree scan. He stood quietly, in plain clothes, but nicely dressed - and ready.

Daniel moved methodically to the counter where the interaction was taking place, and said nothing as he removed his revolver from the back of his jacket and placed it on the counter. The customs agent continued with his barrage of harsh language and threats. He took note of the gun on the counter, and continued his interrogation.

Further intimidation continued and our team member remained quiet and non-confrontational. The tension in the air increased at a constant rate. Again, Daniel said nothing, and slowly with conviction, reached into his pant pocket and pulled out a large bullet, placing it next to the revolver. There was no verbal response from anyone.

The interrogation stopped. Eyes from all sides of the counter were upon the gun and the bullet placed vertically on the counter that accompanied it. The rock was placed back in the duffle by the customs agent, and the zippers were zipped for travel. The gun and the bullet were carefully and slowly placed again in Daniel's jacket for concealment. It was his last means of protection for our team. He had been a remarkable guard, and an outstanding member of our team. Daniel said nothing as he looked at me and returned to his post against the back wall.

Daniel was dear to me, and I hoped that he could return to work with our team. I learned the following year that he was deployed into the Congo on assignment. I hope that someday I will see him again, however, the likelihood of that is very remote. He remained the guard that all would be measured against after his service with our team.

Years passed with guards, men and women who did a good job and many did not come even close to doing well. Guards never measured up to the professional standards and expertise of Daniel, until a couple years ago.

In 2012 there were three guards assigned randomly to our team from the men and women who were serving the country as national police. It was another line up of officers that were ordered to guard our team's travels throughout the Copper Belt region, and into the depths of the tribal bush area.

As the team exited the customs area of the airport, Dr. Henry and I remained behind dealing with the interrogation of the customs officers searching every duffle that we brought in that contained medications. Hours passed as we stood under scrutiny defending the medications, the expiration dates, and the usage of the medications to the customs officers. Every bag was opened, and every bottle, tube, and medical item was examined. Multiple times in the search Henry and I were threatened as to the authenticity of our supplies. It was the norm, but it was not fun or appreciated after a twenty-three-hour flight and nine months of preparation.

We finally passed through the trials and tribulations of customs clearing our drug manifest and exited as always through the gates of the tin airport structure to find my guards assignments lined up and ready for duty.

I gave a quick glance down the row of the assigned officers, accept introductions, and handshake to each, then on to determine which officer would be the most appropriate and professional to be my guard. That person would then be selected to be in charge of the rest of the officers.

I was introduced to the first two officers and then to Detective Sergeant K who, with his stature and response, reflected his professional character and confidence immediately. He reminded me of Daniel in his presentation, but not in appearance. He was a man of very few words, but when he spoke the words seemed profound. His tall muscular frame stood with confidence as his broad shoulders slanted back as he received his position as officer in charge. His handshake was firm, and his voice - baritone - replied, "Madam." He emanated an air of confidence, control, and protection that would guarantee our safety. I had to trust him, as this is how it went each time I entered the country. Intuition and gut reaction was the measuring stick and that's just how it was.

His demeanor was such that, for the first time since Daniel, I addressed him as "Sir", which was awkward in a way for me. He did not ask for that salutation, but his presence seemed to command it. Most other guards were addressed by their surname or their first name depending on the person. This was different.

We had multiple clinics in various locations, some well-known and some new to the team and to me. Derrick spent the days assigned to guard me personally during the clinics and to organize the guards' dismissal at the end of the day and to assemble and have them present each morning before our team set off for another clinic site.

OMNI clinics are new to every officer that moves and travels with us. Crowd control is essential, and our team's safety is paramount in these remote regions. During the clinics, our vehicles have to transport critically ill patients to hospitals, which means having an escort in security accompany them. Vigilance is needed to remove inebriated patients who are disruptive or violent. Personal attention is required to help carry critical patients to triage or beyond. Arrests of criminals, domestic abusers and general safety all is part of their duties.

Our last clinic was in a compound a stone's throw from the Congo border and by all definitions would qualify as a knife and gun club on steroids. There was no law or order, no recognition of time attributing to the drunken stupors starting early in the day. We were providing care under the shadows of a ruthless society who valued no one but themselves. Violence and disorder was the order of the day.

I wanted to test his ability to protect me, perhaps to see if he was as good as I thought he was. I suspect that subconsciously I wanted to see if he was as competent as Daniel was as well. I would watch from my triage station to see when he looked away and would leave my post, slip around the side of the cement building thinking I could make it to the back where I could perhaps walk down a path unnoticed, taking a short walk and then return to the clinic. I never made it beyond the corner, looking back to see a determined, strong and in charge officer, close on my path.

We were set up in a cement block building in another location, and there was a hallway that connected two rooms with the openings in the front, exposed to the crowds waiting outside. I got up and slipped through the back hallway to enter the adjacent room, my only path to move without being seen, and there he was, waiting. I asked, "Can't I go anywhere unattended?"

"No, madam," he replied. "It is my job to watch over you." His vigilance was constant, and I felt protected at all times. I went back to my post of triage and knew that I was not only being watched, but was being protected as well.

Unrest started near sundown as the loud and boisterous village thugs near the Congo border were upset that they had not been fed a meal by our team that day. It was an unusual spot for a clinic, as we had a large electrical tower to the north of the plot and a cinder block building that had "Car Wash" written by hand in white paint. Since there were few cars, and no water, it served as a storefront for coffin making, a thriving business in this part of the world.

We had served over 650 people, had no break and were being chastised by some of the village thugs for not catering to their dietary desires. You could feel the tension in the air, and the atmosphere changed in a matter of a few minutes.

It happened quite rapidly. "We need to leave, pack up the clinic, get the team on the bus, and get in the car," my guard said. As team leader, it was my responsibility to go to each station and give the word that the clinic was closing, and that a rapid tear down was essential. I walked back into the cement barracks that held our pharmacy and our lab.

My instruction to the team was to pack up now, put our meds and supplies into our packs and get to the bus within minutes.

Duffels were packed, tarps that hung as sun blocks were taken down, tables collapsed and loaded, and team members with head lamps adorning their foreheads gathered our belongings onto the bus and its trailer in the shadows of the African dusk.

Derrick lead me to the car and directed me to the back seat. I looked up as he took a final panoramic view of the chaotic crowd, gathering, fires now burning the waste from our clinics and individuals demanding more care. We drove off following the bus and the team until we cleared the compound. Derrick turned to me as we paused on the dirt road, still in view of the compound, with this instruction, "You will not be going back there again." His voice was low, calm, and confident.

I did not argue or respond. I hear you and will listen. His message was stern and I received it knowing that it was his job to protect us. I watched out the window as we drove away. I could see the smoke rising from the recently built fire that we started to burn the clinic waste. The scene behind us looked like the edge of a war zone.

We left behind us the bordering village to the Congo, complete with thugs, violence, unrest, and disrespect. We left unattended needs, children who had no access to medical care, and mothers who needed help. Smoke rose from the beginning of ashes of the fires that were burning. Electrical towers loomed over the car wash that no one used. Smoke filled the clinic area where patients once stood earlier in the day.

Prostitution, men who controlled the young girls, and greed stood in the shadows of the border town. The silhouette was hazy in our rear view mirrors. My heart ached at the thought of not finishing our clinic to serve those in need. My mind, however, realized that my guard was doing an amazing job at protecting us. We drove on.

Derrick's strong presence and professional character was apparently instilled in him by his father who was also a well-respected and a tenured high ranking officer within the Zambian national police force. His father groomed him from an early age to be a man of integrity, striving always to be of good character and disciplined by honesty and commitment.

I had the opportunity to meet him at the local police station, where he stood outside the building waiting for our vehicle to arrive. We had come in the middle of the day to check on the deployment of an officer for the next day. Derrick's father presented like a man of great strength, wisdom and confidence. He stood tall and looked very strong in his physical presence and his confidence. We shook hands and he and Derrick greeted each other warmly and with mutual respect. I was honored to meet him and could see the resemblance in these two fine men, who possessed a rare quality of esteemed gentle giants among us.

Back at our lodge that evening, Joshua showed up unannounced and wanting to speak to me. He had been coming to our clinics over the years and helping us with interpretation. Each time, however, he managed to leave with money that he had begged for from team members and me for various needs. I had paid for his high school for four years and had found a sponsor to send him through college for nurses training in the capital. Despite all of the support, he always wanted and asked for more. His requests became very dramatic and at times demanding. Politely but firmly, we supported his needs for school, transportation, and clothing.

My family sponsored Joshua to attend four years at a private school run by the British. I also provided money for his uniforms, food, and transportation. Once he finished high school and graduated, he had been gifted with an education that very few in that region could ever obtain.

Joshua was persistent in his desire for an education. Unable to continue his support, OMNI offered to find a sponsor for him, and, within a few weeks, a kind woman, who also valued education, offered to send him to college in Zambia. Three years later, he finished the nursing program, however, he did not obtain a degree. Reasons for this were unclear.

Two years later, a local practicing member of witchcraft murdered Joshua's father not far from Agape Farm. Eventually, Joshua inherited the vast verdant land that his father once owned, and, now, is one of the largest land owners in that area. We continue to hear from him each time the team comes into the country, and he volunteers at the clinics.

The following day our team was back at Baluba, the Congolese refugee village that is very near to the border of the Congo. Our first patient of the day had just delivered her first baby three days earlier and was now running a high fever, had a very high pulse and was breathing rapidly and with shallow breathes.

Dr. Henry examined her finding a ridged abdomen, tenderness, and distention indicating perhaps a postpartum infection. Her pulse seemed thready as we continued our history intake of her and it was determined rather quickly that she needed to be admitted into the hospital.

Derrick carried her and placed her in the back seat of our vehicle and Andrew, a pre-med student who was also an EMT, got into the back of the car to accompany her to the hospital some thirty minutes away.

"She is getting worse," I said. "Please drive fast. I feel she is going to go into shock from sepsis," I added.

We sped out of the compound down a dirt road miles away from the main road. We discussed a plan of how we would provide CPR on her in the back seat despite the cramped space that was for the three of us. Derrick was now making it to the main road and the speedometer exceeded eighty-five as we wove through the maze of traffic, passing large semis heading south from the Congo.

The ride was frightening as the situation of this young woman becoming septic and she was going into shock. We approached the roundabout and I had to tell Derrick to slow way down, or none of us would make it to the hospital at this dangerous speed and with the congested traffic.

We approached the armed checkpoint and Derrick waved to them allowing us to pass without being stopped. We pulled up into the emergency room parking lot and found an old metal gurney to place our patient on and wheel her into the waiting area. People lined the narrow halls sitting on the wooden benches waiting to be seen, some two and three deep. There seemed to be no movement of the lines.

Our team shirts and stethoscopes seemed to allow us access into the small room where six gurneys were lined against the dark walls filled with critically ill patients. I was not sure that all of them were alive as one man appeared to have passed. Stained, worn cloth curtains hung from metal bars that, when pulled, allowed some visual privacy, but one could hear moans and voices from each patient.

I went to the paper cluttered desk that sat in the middle of the room and located who appeared to be the receiving physician and introduced myself, and offered my card for identification. OMNI was received with appreciation for the work that we were doing and our patient was examined within a few minutes. Fortunately, for her, she was admitted directly to the gynecological floor where and IV and antibiotics were started.

Our diagnoses was correct and without our care this young mother would have died, leaving another baby orphaned in Baluba. We drove back to the clinic site, maintaining the speed now of the surrounding traffic as there were over 500 patients waiting to be seen.

We were only back to work a few minutes and another emergency case came walking to the head of the line accompanied by her husband and two small children. She held her hand over her eyes and was unable to open them because of the severe pain she was experiencing.

My history report for this young woman read:

"Thirty-two-year-old ambulatory female complaining of pain in both eyes, was working in her garden ten minutes ago when a cobra spit in the eyes. Patient accompanied by husband and children. Complaining of diminishing, cloudy site. Husband killed snake with the garden hoe before leaving for the clinic."

Our emergency trauma doctor examined her and ordered copious amounts of water for flushing out both eyes for thirty minutes, and to take and record her vital signs every ten minutes. I used our team water and poured a steady stream over her eyes monitoring her blood pressure and pulse frequently. She started to complain about feeling

307

warm, and I asked her to stay still while I got the doctor back to check her. When we returned a few minutes later, she and her family were gone. We were unable to find her in the crowd and prayed that she would survive and keep her sight.

Shortly after the completion of our clinics, the team prepared our departure from the country when I said my goodbyes to the staff and the guards. "Thank you for protecting me, and for your fine professional care," I said as we were leaving. "You remind me of someone," I said to Derrick. "His name is Daniel, and I didn't think I would find another guard like him." I didn't think that I would see him again, but wanted to compliment him on his work that week for our team.

A few months later, I was back in the country on business and requested to have Derrick as my personal guard. It was a long shot, as guards are rarely used twice for our team. The pay and the experience of being with OMNI assist and supplement each officer's salary, and so their officers in charge spread out the assignments so that all men and women can benefit. But this time, we were blessed with a repeat assignment. We were in country to dedicate the opening of the Morgan Harrington Educational Wing and our guest of honor was the former First Lady of the country, Dr. Maureen Mwanawasa. Our security must be experienced, excelling in professional attention and details. Our group was to be honored by her presence for dinner the night before and she had accepted our invitation to stay overnight in a private suite in our lodge.

Derrick accepted his assignment to be my guard and to be present that evening for the dinner honoring the First Lady of Zambia. It was a beautiful evening in December, and the staff at the lodge had prepared a special meal, and set a table for us under the stars of Africa, complete with a few bottles of fine South African wines.

He secured the west wing of the lodge for its safety and for secure perimeters as it was where the First Lady would stay just down the hall from our room. Her room had to be checked prior to her arrival, flowers placed on the table next to her bed, and a tray with hot tea, bottled water and biscuits were prepared by the staff.

Her personal bodyguard accompanied her to her room to secure her safety, and then left to remain ready at her car should she need to be driven anywhere. Dinner was lovely and the conversation was global and lively. I sat to the First Lady's right, with our backs to the wall, strategically placed so that he could see the grounds and all entrances. First ladies are always served first and their glasses and plates removed first. She was elegant and classy, yet down to earth and warm in her reception of us. The night was lovely in all ways.

Prior to her retirement to her room, the west wing was once again checked, and Derrick escorted her to her room, and then me to mine. His professionalism was remarkable and he carried out his duties with confidence. Safe and secure, we were all locked in for the night.

Chriss and Gil and I shared a room and could discuss the evening and all of the details once we were in our rooms. It had been a wonderful night filled with amazing stories of the First Lady and her time with her husband while he was the president of Zambia. It was clear that she missed him very much since his death a few years earlier.

I had brought a gift for the First Lady knowing that she would be our guest on the women's wing of the lodge. Before her retirement to her room just a few steps down the hall from Chriss, Gil, and me. I presented her with a lounge set and chocolates fit for a First Lady. She seemed genuinely happy to receive the gift and mentioned something about it feeling like Christmas. I was pleased to know that we were so well received by her as her company over the years has been that of royalty and dignitaries from all over the world. We were just the girls and were enjoying this unique experience.

Interestingly enough, this First Lady was the owner of Setanga Lodge, the very home to OMNI when we were in country. The lodge was originally a private home located just blocks behind the city cemetery, walking distance through two other private homes and yards.

The L-shaped structure had rooms down the hall to the right, two rooms across the back yard large enough for a double bed and a night stand, and adjacent to a pool that was always full of green water. On most trips, the pool had only a few feet of water at the deep end which was an ever deeper shade of swamp green. Care must be taken when maneuvering around the pool at night if you drew the short straw for the poolside rooms.

A beautiful small guest house stood across from the one stall carport and had three rooms and one bath. It also had a bonus room of a tiny kitchen complete with a refrigerator and sink. The water pressure and reliability of water was less than "iffy" on both sides. A guard dog roamed the grounds and Guinea hens scattered from bush to bush, using their obnoxious wake up calls at 4:30 a.m. to all enclosed in the property.

Local residents made up the staff. They walked to the grounds daily, kept us happy with amazing hearty meals such as chicken, beef, and many delicious vegetables - raw, roasted, and grilled. On the most wonderful days, we would arrive home to a meal in the making and a chocolate cake baked just that afternoon.

Most of the time, however, we entered a dark site. Power shedding is common in Ndola and one never knows when the government or the surrounding country of Congo will use the power. We had to be prepared with headlamps, and if fortunate, single candles were lit in the dining area.

No power meant a later than usual dinner, as food was cooked over a fire in the backyard over an open pit. An oil drum split in half and fit with iron bars made for the most amazing outdoor fire pit. Chicken and vegetables on those nights were the best.

No power also means no water. After a fourteen-hour day in the bush and treating the diseases of the world, a face and hand washing was desperately needed. We caught on as time when on and planned ahead of time by filling the bathtubs in the girls' wing with water so that we could dip a cup into it and wash our hands and face. Unknown to us, and unannounced, the lights sometimes would come on late at night or, even better, in the middle of the night. Cheers could be heard from rooms all over the small lodge that we called home.

We unloaded the forty fifty-pound duffels into the carport and each night would go out with headlamps and rearrange the items needed for the next clinic. Staff encouraged our team members to help before baths or dinner could be had. It was our evening ritual before we debriefed and talked about the challenges of the day. Those debriefings were

often times painful and encouraging. Highs and lows were exchanged along with prayers for those who experienced the lows that the day offered. The lows usually were described as a child or an adult who had been diagnosed with a life ending disease, and there was little that we could do other than pray for them. In the end, that is the gift beyond what they had and we were comforted by that.

Because this was a small local lodge, and I do mean small, we had to often times share our space with others who were working in Zambia or in bordering countries.

Steve was such that man, and we shared a space and common dining area with him on many evenings and many years. He lived at Setanga. A young man from Canada, Stan arrived in Africa to work with a drilling company excavating for diamonds and gems in the Congo. Each morning, he would start up his truck just outside of my small room and head to the Congo border for work.

Since there were no window panes in my bedroom, the diesel exhaust from his truck filled my room each morning with a pungent odor. Noise from the engine and the equipment being loaded into the truck served as my wakeup call. On one of his daily trips, he noticed a stray dog, hungry, and alone. Stan was alone as well, having left his parent and family behind to seek adventure on an unknown continent to him. He took the dog home in his truck and named him "Congo." They were inseparable and both needed each other more than they were willing to admit.

Once across the border, Stan let Congo out of the truck so he could run along the side of the truck in the bush area as he had been accustomed to do. The turn to the left came suddenly, and Stan's front truck tire crushed Congo underneath. Not to leave his buddy behind, Stan loaded him into the truck and brought him back to the lodge where he recovered for several weeks before his return to duty. Congo remained loyal to Stan and Stan to him.

Stan drank heavily each night, in attempts to drown painful memories from his past, and perhaps to numb the dangerous life that he was now living. At the small bar in the gathering area, and after many local beers, Stan told his story.

"My buddy and I crossed every day into the Congo, working on the rigs and coming home at night. The money is good, but the dangers far exceed the money. We decided to shorten our travel one day and crossed over the border on an unmarked and unmanned road into the Congo. We were caught and brought to the nearest village by the border police." He continued his story of that fateful crossing, describing the porous border between Congo and Zambia.

"We were brought to the village center and told to stand under the flagpole. They put a gun to our heads and warned us never to cross over again or they would kill us. I have never been so afraid in my life. The interrogation lasted for a couple of hours. I thought that we might be able to leave after they made their point. We agreed, and, for the life of me, I don't know why I was spared. I thought we could both leave." His voice quivered, "they shot my buddy in the head right in front of me, and then let me go." He took another drink of his beer and asked for another. The ashtray in front of him was filling with beer caps from the local brew.

"I was allowed to leave in my truck, leaving my buddy dead on the ground. I was told that, when I passed over the border each day, I had to bring fresh loaves of bread to the border guards or I would end up like my buddy. I leave early now each day and load my truck with fresh bread to leave at the border. I don't know when it will be enough."

His face was red with alcohol and the heat of the day. His eyes were bloodshot and intense as he looked away.

He spoke of his family in Canada and how much he missed seeing his mother. He had not seen anyone in a couple of years. It was clear that he was hurting despite his tough-looking exterior. His alcohol consumption was high every night, and he often times kept company with women who worked the streets, targeting men just like him.

After that night, the sound of his truck starting reminded me of the dangers they faced that none of us could imagine.

Years later, we found out that Stan had been shot and killed in a hotel room in Johannesburg while purchasing the sexual favors from a prostitute. His life ended tragically on the heels of a dangerous and risky lifestyle in Africa, working as a driller in the Congo.

At the same small lodge, we shared common space with a man who kept to himself occasionally walking through and greeting us with a short grunt of a hello. His quarters for sleeping were in a single tiny room off of the car port. I never saw him when he was not drunk or attempting to balance a cigarette from the opposite hand that held his drink. He too worked in the Congo as a driller. His skin was worn and weathered and his heavy British accent was almost hard to understand mingled in with his drunken stupor. He was lonely and often times rambled on in our presence before he retired to his modest quarters. It seemed like a pathetic existence, and could not understand how any amount of money would be worth this pain.

One night, after we had all retired to our rooms, locked our doors and prayed that we would not be bit in the night by mosquitos, the noise across the courtyard at our lodge kept me awake. I slept under the open window in a small single bed just to the left inside of the room that I shared with two other nurses on our team.

"Let me tell you this story that will amaze you," one of them said.

"Well only if you will let me tell you what I did today," said the second one.

Laughter, knee slapping and hand slaps to the counter followed each story. There were multiple offers to buy each man another drink of which they did.

"You bought the last one," said the first one.

"I know but I want to buy this one," said the second one.

Laughter after each garbled story continued until nearly 1 a.m.

I thought, *Will these guys ever go to bed so that we can sleep? We have to get up in a few hours and take care of another 600 people, and we need our sleep!*

I pulled back the thin curtain clouding the view from my room to the tiny counter that housed the late party and found one man. Several beer bottles were scattered around the small counter and the ashtray was full of spent cigarettes. In observation, he was two voices, two personalities haphazardly trapped in one worn body.

316

Working in the Congo does crazy things to these poor men, I thought. *At least he is never alone!* His party ended and the two personalities retired to their room. It was 2 a.m. and we had to get up in a few hours to start our work. I had to get some sleep as the patient load the next day was anticipated to be heavy.

Up at six a.m., breakfast at 7 a.m., load the bus with the day's ration of medications and supplies, then down to join the others. Large five-gallon portable travel jugs were filled with water from our bath tub since it was too heavy to lift down from the sink. The tetanus had been kept on dry ice overnight to preserve it and Gil kept that little red tote close to her supplies and marked.

We picked up cases of water for the team and for the pharmacy to fill the antibiotic suspensions and hydration packet for those that were suffering from malaria of other tropical diseases. Each team member was given a small power bar to eat at some point during the day. I never seemed to be able to take the time to eat all of mine except for a bite or two. The rest was almost always given to some child that I had triaged who needed it far greater than me. I could always eat at night when we got back to the lodge. They would go home to nothing.

We worked past sun down again, closing the clinic in the pitch dark with head lamps and small flash lights. We medically served over 600 patients that day. We worked from sun up to sun down and were exhausted, but loved every minute of it. There was roasted chicken on the grill when we got back to the lodge and local greens cooking in the pot. We were fortunate that day that they also had roasted potatoes that day. Nothing ever smelled or tasted so good especially when you have worked all day and had not eaten for fifteen hours.

We took turns using the showers and hoped that there was enough hot water left for the last few people. I always had work to tend to for the next day or had a meeting with someone who 'just wanted a minute of my time'. I drew the last in line for the showers and the hot water was again long gone. I've learned that water at any temperature whether for bathing or drinking in Africa is a blessing. Far too many nights, the electricity was out when we returned, and so was the water. A bottle of water becomes the source for getting clean, and I appreciated that too.

Separated by just a couple of months, the business trip shortly followed after the medical trip that year. At our school, just a few miles from where the team was staying, the first graduating class was about to accept their certificates and to launch into the next phase of their life. Thirteen young girls and boys made up the class. They were the product of hard work, a vision for the poor and God's blessings. They were making history in the village as the first children to graduate from the seventh grade.

I had carried over green shiny graduation gowns and hats complete with a gold tassel for each graduate. The primary green color was a prominent shade in the Zambian flag and represented growth and life in these amazing children. Each child proudly received his or her gown and quickly went into one of the rooms at the school to try it on. You could palpate the excitement in the room.

Grace was one of our oldest graduates, reaching twenty years as she approached her graduation. I so admired her for her determination and her ability to triumph over adversity. Grace was born with a severe congenital hip that created shortness in her right leg causing her spine to curve like the letter "S". It resembles scoliosis but the origin was definitely coming from her deteriorating hip. For her to walk took a great deal of effort as her gate was exaggerated and cumbersome. She often had to sit or lean against a building to take the weight and stress off of her spine and hip.

There was always a smile on her face despite the pain her little body endured. The day before the graduation, Grace was determined to participate along with her classmates in the rehearsal performance which required her to walk down the dirt path from the security gate, to building one and down the path that was created by the rented metal chairs. Her seat was in the front row and just to the right of the isle.

I watched as the students came in, each of them dancing to the national music that was blaring from the small boom box in the front of the chairs. She was clearly in pain, but managed to walk in with her class. Grace offered no complaints although she had the right to do so.

Dr. Jim and I were there to watch the students come in. Jim was especially drawn to her case because of his orthopedic expertise. Jim met with Grace's parents and promised to come back and operate on Grace and give her a new hip, and correct the spinal anomaly.

We had hope for Grace. Her father had hope and most importantly, Grace had hope that someone would help her to gain a life without pain and physical struggles.

The day before the ceremony was as emotional as the day of the event. One of our students was pregnant, and one of our male students admitted to fathering the child.

Our policy in the school was that sexual conduct between students would lead to immediate expulsion. It was a policy that had been put in place to protect our students and to provide a boundary of appropriate behavior in the remote tribal region.

I had signed the policy for good reason and now was faced with two students who had worked hard, were bright, and had been given a chance of hope for the future. They were both brought before me the morning of the rehearsal so that I could repeat the policy and terminate their position at the OMNI School, just one day prior to their graduation.

The meeting was done in a small room with the headmaster, two board members, and Derrick representing security. The young man came in first and I fully expected to see a defiant and indignant boy before me. After I read the policy to him and spoke about the actions that he had taken, I had to dismiss him, pulling him from the graduation ceremony, in accordance to our policy.

"Thank you, madam. I am grateful for all that OMNI has done for me and my family," he said. "Just being able to participate in the graduation practice is enough for me as I would have never been able to do even this without OMNI's help."

He got up and with his head low, shook all of our hands before exiting the room.

The young girl came in next. The tiny baby that she had delivered just two weeks ago was being held by her sister just outside the school building. She was a mother now, and seemed well beyond her short seventeen years. Her acknowledgment of her pregnancy and the lack of focus on her studies were profound. She was polite, remorseful and
appreciative of her education. She was very quiet, keeping her eyes low in respect of authority and left the room once our conversation was over.

I was heartbroken for them and so sad that neither one of them would be allowed to participate in the formal graduation in the morning. Tears welled up and my heart was very heavy. I didn't sleep well that night thinking about the boy, the girl, and the baby. Their chance at a future seemed to have been thwarted with the policy that we had in place.

Before the festivities started I called an emergency meeting of the board members that were present to discuss the termination of the two students and their expulsion from the graduation ceremonies. My question to them was this: "What would Jesus have done now? Would he turn his back, or make this a moment of grace in the form of an extended olive branch? Where do we stand firm on policy and where does compassion and wisdom come in?" The OMNI board was silent and then Jim and Mary Sue spoke, "We were hoping and praying that this question would be asked and that these students could graduate with their class. They made mistakes, but were remorseful and showed such appreciation for their education. Despite their expulsion, both came and participated the rehearsal and in the clean-up of the day."

It was true. I watched them both, and neither had any animosity toward our decision and worked hard to stack the chairs, clean up and participate despite knowing they would not be allowed to walk with their class. More amazing to all of us, was that they did all of this with a smile on their face and a terrific attitude. We were proud of them and of their choice to be grateful for what they had at that moment.

The decision was unanimous to allow them both to graduate and participate fully in all of the ceremonies and activities of the day. It was a decision that each of us felt good about making.

I called them both in before the caps and gowns were distributed and told them of our decision to allow them to graduate with their class because of their amazing attitude and behavior through this very difficult time. Both of them got up from their chairs and extended their hand to greet me. I hugged them both and knew that they had learned more at this moment in life than the last seven years. Compassion once given will send of ripples for generations to come.

Kevin recognizes me from time to time as we travel along the dirt road to the OMNI School. I always ask for the truck to stop so that I can greet him. The bond is a solid one of mutual respect and appreciation. No words need to be spoken when we greet. I am proud of him and know that he will grow to be a good man.

Derrick coordinated the guards who attended the gate, the grounds and the vehicles that delivered the First Lady to our site. His leadership and management skills were quite apparent especially on this high level of security. Our armed guards were walking the grounds watching all entrances and the perimeter. The First Lady's guard was attending to her safety and security. Derrick kept an eye on me and our team. I felt safe but uneasy with one of our prominent employees missing on such an important day.

The grounds had to be continually checked every fifteen minutes and armed guards were situated on the perimeter of our property for additional security. Having the First Lady there increased our responsibility and we understood the importance of this requirement. The ceremony was going well, however, Anton had still not shown up and we had to scramble with little time left to set up the chairs and bring the sound equipment. Our team members had to take one of our trucks and go and pick up the equipment which really made everyone scramble to get the work done. Our vehicle had been missing since the day before and we suspected that he had been driving that as well. His absence was troublesome and showed how totally irresponsible he was.

The graduation ceremony was to honor those students and their achievements and to dedicate our new school building. Mothers, hair combed and wrapped in traditional fabric matching their dresses walked down the dusty dirt road to the school to witness their first graduation. Siblings and other family members walked in and sat in the hot sun waiting for the ceremony to begin. The chairs that we rented filled quickly and a crowd of over 400 parents, dignitaries, students, staff, and government representatives attended.

The music began and the thirteen who had all passed their final exams and efficiency tests joined the processional, in a dance, march like entrance. As soon as the students could be seen in their bright green gowns, the mothers of the students started trilling, clapping and dancing. Tradition allowed them to dance forward and join their son or daughter and proceed with them until they reached their chairs in the front.

Teddy and the teachers marched in the procession and the same mothers ran forward and adorned them with the scarves that they had around their neck, placing them on his shoulders. This gesture indicated their high respect and appreciation for the hard work that he had done with their children over the years. The moment was epic and historic and I watched as a dream of mine became a reality. Orphan, vulnerable children products of extreme poverty were coming forward to receive their certification of education. Each could read, write, do math, know geography, knew their sciences and were the first in their community to escape the downward spiral of poverty and its grasps.

We watched the students with a great deal of pride. I was also watching my periphery and wondered where our director and our car were located. Both were four hours late.

As the ceremony took place, and guest speakers, and our teachers presented their messages of congratulations, our vehicle stopped at the outside security gate and motioned to the guards to be let in. It slowly drove over to the left side of the campus with our employee inside and parked near the administration building. Anton emerged having on the same clothes as the day before. Instead of arriving in the dress suit that was planned his work clothes were quite disheveled and dirty. He was staggering and apparently intoxicated.

The First Lady of the country was sitting to my left and was focused on the current speaker. I motioned to Derrick to check out the situation of which he already had his eyes on. He circled around to take the keys from him and I could see that a discussion and interrogation was taking place. Derrick asked him to wait to have a discussion with me after the ceremony. The First Lady was our priority, our 400 guests, and eventually this problem would be addressed.

The ceremony went on and after a large dinner for the guests and the First Lady, people started to leave the area to go home. The board members and I had a brief meeting and after an intense discussion about employee behavior and violation of policies had to terminate the man that came in four hours late and drunk. The discussion that continued far too long included a wild story of how the employee had been chased the night before by road bandits, causing him to drive for hours, finally ending up in a road side hotel in Baluba. The story, the mileage, the scenario that was presented could only have been fabricated and did not match the facts that we knew. The fuel and odometer readings did not match the length of the so called route, and the story became bigger than life, and the inebriation coupled with changing recollections deemed to be unfortunately false. It was the end of the road for this employee, and there was no other way to handle it.

As the week came to an end, so was his duty to guard our team and me. I knew that we would not be able to hire him again as we had already extended his tour with us more than the allotted time. I thought of his rare qualities and his strong character that I respected. I hoped that he possessed the integrity that we were looking for in a permanent member of our organization. As we had been burned before and especially just the day before proceeding forward with another employee had to be taken with caution.

I took it before of my board members who were present on the trip. The men and women of the OMNI board of directors are hand chosen and have sound character, wisdom and impeccable integrity.

Doug listened and had observed the actions of Derrick as well. He gave his endorsement to hire Derrick, and the next step would be up to me.

I met with Derrick that afternoon privately at the lawn chairs near our lodge and asked if he would be interested in leaving the police force and taking a position with OMNI. I felt that it was a long shot on my part, knowing that he came from a strong family background of law enforcement. In harmony with his character, he replied to my offer, "I want to lie down with my wife, and seek her opinion and then discuss this with my father of whom I respect."

I was pleased to hear that he would also seek advice and feedback before taking such a position. It showed his strong character and respect of his family. I found this to be another attribute to his integrity.

The following morning Derrick returned, dressed in a suit and accepted the position as my personal guard, and Director of Human Resources with OMNI. He would attend classes for his business degree at the same time, and would take a leave from his previous position with the national police. His father gave his blessing to take a leave from the police force and take up this position, which later would be an important milestone in his life. Giving the blessing to leave a post that emulated his father's success was notable on both sides.

A few months later, news broke across the international news headlines of a fatal crash in Zambia taking the lives of an entire bus load of people traveling south from Ndola to the capital. I read about it online and again learned more on international news stations. An email followed shortly from the headmaster of my school of the news. Derrick's distinguished, remarkable and iconic father died in a fatal car accident along with several other people that day along the road near Kabwe. There was only one lone survivor in more than thirty passengers. His loss was devastating to the community, the police force, and the entire country, most especially to his son Derrick.

Derrick traveled to the site of the crash on behalf of the family to identify his father's body and had to be the one to deliver the news to his mother. Upon arrival, he was asked to walk through the makeshift morgue and pass multiple bodies before he would reach the most important man in his life. Identification was made, and to Derrick's horrible reality, was the death of his beloved father. Ironically, as though it was a gift given to both, Derrick's father had placed a phone call connecting them to each other as the vehicle was struck. Two remarkable men, each a protector in society. Each man is and was absolutely astonishing.

Security at our site is a twenty-four-hour necessity, with guards during the day, and a change to armed guards at night. The addition of armed guards occurred after a break in one evening in the early hours of the night shift. A gang of five or six men with wire cutters broke into our compound, and using force, tied up our guards, forcing them to stay face down onto the dirt. Pedro tried to look up and see who the perpetrators were and was beaten with a metal pipe, breaking his ankle and inflicting a head wound resulting in a concussion. Our other guard was beaten and held down, both unable to get up.

They stole computers, electronics and items from the school that could be easily sold on the streets for cash. Reports were filed, and Derrick was in charge of following up on the case. Weeks went by until I was back in the country and asked for a report on the case and the men who stole from us. It was found that the men were from a village distant to ours, and had a history of theft and violence. I asked Derrick for an update when I entered the country. "Madam, I have taken care of it," he said.

"And..." My sentenced stopped as I knew Derrick would need little more prompting than that. He remained with his composure and with his assurance of what he knew and had been trained to do.

"Well, I tracked three of them down, shot one in the knee, one in the hip, and I wrestled the other to the ground. It took a while, but I got them Madam," he confidently and without hesitation replied. "They were arrested and are in jail." I learned that the other men were still being sought after to this day. They perhaps have learned not to mess with Derrick.

He made it sound easy, and reports in a calm and matter-of-fact manner. I suspected that it must have been quite an episode, of which Derrick was more than capable of taking care of.

Amazing, I thought. *Absolutely amazing.* Physical strength and courage, and years of training that through strategy and planning apprehended these men.

With equal parts of strength and courage, there remain the same qualities of compassion and gentleness. I have seen Derrick hold a tiny child in the clinics trying to comfort them, and kneeling down in front of an old man out of respect for his position as an elder.

There have been many times, when threats do not come in the form of physical violence, but posturing and intimidation. It is an interesting form of control, or attempt of it. If one was intimidated, one would back down and lose the mind game. Derrick was not of that make. When confronted by a man that attempted to overpower him, by intimidation, the outcome was predictable knowing the confidence and self-control that he possesses.

"I am a bear!" shouted the angry man that was working on our property as he pointed his finger at Derrick. It was an attempt to show control and the adult version of bullying. It was clear that this man chose an animal that he felt would intimidate Derrick into complying with his demands.

"I am a lion!" came his response in his deep and calm voice.

Lions used to roam through the great Savanna that divides the deep bush with its golden grass and African sunsets. Lions are symbols of strength and courage and have been celebrated throughout history for these characteristics. They symbolize wisdom, power, dignity, courage, justice, ferocity and dominion. The conversation ended, and the lion walked away with confidence. The bear, was intimidated, turned and walked away and took cover. It was not to show its teeth again as his intimidation was not effective.

Later when Derrick, Teddy, and I was walking the fence line of our property he told the following story to me as we stopped in the shade under a mango tree.

"I am Derrick Musakanya Kalinda, known in my family as King White Lion.

"According to the tradition here in Zambia every tribe has clans of people with a particular culture and beliefs example is abena mfula (rain), which means the rains representing them, abena nshimu, the bees represent them, abena Mumba (Name of a person) a name which represents a certain group of people just to name a few and the lion (abena nkalamu), which represents my clan.

"Just a brief explanation on how people or persons were named after animals, trees, rains or water was like this, Abena Mumba is a reality situation that happened a long time ago, there was famine in that land and only one family called the Mumba family had enough food stored at their house and the entire village knew about the Mumba's," he said.

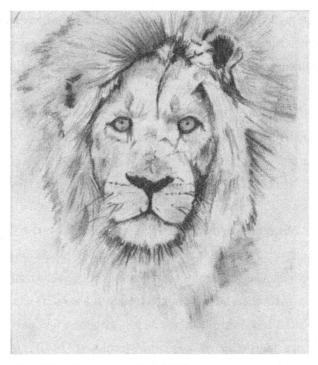

Pencil Sketch by Karen R. ReMine

He went on to explain: "This family could receive a lot of visitors only during lunch time when eating as the people used to hide in the bushes watching at a distance if the cooking was completed and then show up. The Mumba's family observed that people were hiding by the nearby bushes so they decided to cut down the trees to the height reaching the knees of a person. The same evenings during dinner and all was set everybody inside the hut where they used to have meals from and before starting to eat. They decided to look around to check if anybody was turning up to join them uninvited and ended up seeing the cut down tree thinking that someone was already hiding and they had to hide the food and waited all night without eating."

Derrick went on to say, "Abena Nkalamu, which is a clan represented by the lion, the people who were named after the lion because of their characteristics of being very strong, hardworking, born leaders, and helpful to strangers by giving them food and where to sleep during night time.

"My middle name is called Musakanya," said Derrick, "which means a white lion which the people believed was a spiritual lion. It only appeared to chosen ones, the chosen people of the land. Musakanya is a name given to the Kings of the Bisa speaking people of the Bemba of Northern Province of Zambia.

"To this present time a mountain in the northern part of the country is named Musakanya Kombe which is near Mpika Boys secondary school were the lion used to appear and leaders of the land could take gifts and offerings and during evening time they could hear the lion roaming.

"Kalinda means the protector or caretaker. Throughout my life since childhood I have been chosen a leader. When I was in grade one was a class captain until grade seven, grade eight to grade nine, I was chosen prefect at Mitobo basic school, grade ten to twelve, I was chosen prefect at St John's convent high school in Kitwe, During my training as a police officer at Kamfinsa police training school I was chosen as the overall squad leader among 475 recruits and nineteen squads, which had twenty-five members each and instructor, at Twapia police station chosen as leader in the criminal investigations department unit as C.I.O and currently at Omni as Director Human Resource. This shows that indeed am a lion born leader and protector among the peoples of the land."

"Indeed, Derrick," I said, "You are the lion, astonishing protector among the people of the land."

Baluba: Surviving the Storm

Our medical team returned the following July to start our mobile medical clinics in the tribal regions. With every trip in, our physicians, and nurses have to be licensed in the country each year. This year was no different, and so shortly after landing in Zambia after a two-day flight, Gil and I had to purchase a ticket on a small commuter plane to fly from Ndola to the Capital that afternoon to present before the nursing council in the morning. Derrick would fly with us for protection and we would all be back in the morning after our appointment.

The flight for Gil and I was pretty routine, having flown many times over many years in various sizes of airplanes and jets. For Derrick, this would be his first flight ever and you could see the anticipation on his face as we boarded the tiny aircraft around eighteen hours for the one-hour flight south.

The smaller plane held about twelve of us, the pilot and a stewardess. Once the engines started the noise level was very high so conversation was difficult. As we taxied down the runway, the stewardess made an announcement at the top of her voice that we were not flying directly to the capital but had been asked to fly to the eastern jungle region near the Zimbabwe border to pick up two people who had been stranded there when their aircraft had broken down. The flight would take us two hours out of our way, and then another two hours to our destination of the capital.

Gil and I just smiled and knew that we were back in Africa, and reminded ourselves that "Plan A" never works. This was "Plan B" and who knew how many more alternative routes would be ahead of us.

This was not your typical flight, but Derrick seemed to enjoy it and was trying to be comfortable in the very small aisle seat that was just wide enough for a small person of which he is not. We flew east then landed and sat on the tiny runway as the next passengers were arranging themselves also for this unscheduled flight. It was dark now and I really could not tell where we were. We had been flying now for three days since we left DC, and I was ready to get out.

We arrived in the capital four hours later than originally expected, and our hotel had decided that we were a no show. The taxi driver took us through a winding route through impoverished compounds and indirect routes. It reminded me of a scary taxi ride in Calcutta, India years ago that took on a dangerous feel to it. After many questions and unnecessary detours, we finally arrived at a hotel where we would stay for the night in preparation for our meeting in the morning.

We made our appointment, obtained our license once again, and caught the 11 a.m. flight back to the Copper Belt region to meet our team. The clinic had already started and we went right to work. The lines were long and the medical team was happy to see our return to fortify the group. We worked past sundown, and closed the clinic for the first night in head lamps. Gil and I were happy to finally get to the lodge where we would catch a quick few hours of sleep before we headed out in the morning to Baluba.

She sat on the cold gray cement block near the end of the building that was intended for a school. It was the first patient of the day at Baluba, the Congolese refugee village, near the Congo border. Chriss ran to me across the compound and said I should check on her first despite the 400 plus people that were in line to be seen by our medical team. Her eyes were cast downward and her body was slight as though she had tried to shrink into a state that would be less noticeable by any perpetrator.

She sat alone on the cold surface and was frail, fragile and broken of spirit. I knelt down in order to see her face as she would not lift her head enough to view the full surface of her face. Her left eye was deep red, swollen around the orbit and blackened by an obvious blow of force. We helped her up to stand up, yet her stature was diminished not by ability, but by fragility of the abuse.

Our exam room was the same room that Holten had died in the year before. The same room that two women lay on the floor next to him near death from malaria. It was the same room that heaven seemed to reach down from the sky and meet the soles that lay there waiting to be relieved from their suffering.

The village or the setting had not changed. The building was more worn, and perhaps there was a slight bit more graffiti than last year. The extreme poverty level remained constant and so were the medical and physical needs of the people who struggled to live there. Babies had been born and people had died in our absence as life here was challenging and at times lethal. The large tree in the center of the field in front of the building provided constant shade from the intense African sun, and the villagers found one of the only comforts there that this village had to offer.

Inside the cement block building, the walls held the damp cold from the night before, and as I knelt down to this woman, I remembered the cold floor from kneeling over Holten as he died. I visualized his frail body taking his last breath in the same location that we were now. Focusing on her face, I could no longer feel the cold, and could no longer hear the crowds of people waiting outside for care.

I asked her to sit down on the rugged bench that was our only piece of furniture in the room. There was no electricity and despite it being early morning, there was little light to see this beautiful woman's battered face. Her eye was a deep red where the white should have been and despite her dark brown skin, the not so beautiful colors of blue and purple were replacing her natural color.

Dr. Henry was called to exam her as I stood near her, somewhat wanted to protect her from further abuse and at the same time wanting to seek all information to document another abuse case in an ever increasing atmosphere of violence against women. Through my personal guard now acting as an interpreter, she admitted that the blow to her face was the result of her husband's fist slamming against her face in his fit of rage last week.

She reluctantly reported that he was drunk and in his state of alcoholic rage, hit her face, and punched her in the ribs. Upon exam, she was shattered - ribs broken on both sides, and her cheekbones had been crushed. She was posed in the classic stature of a downward glance, too broken to be stately any longer. Her ten-month old baby was in line with a family member who was trying to protect them both by coming to our clinic for help.

Although this was our first case of the early morning in Baluba, it was not our last of domestic violence. It was the sample of how the day would unfold, in bursts of dysfunctional relationships and advanced diseases.

Derrick was quick to respond to my request for law enforcement involvement, and another officer on our team was called to take a statement. The presence of a nurse, a physician, and two armed guards created a team of support for her that she had perhaps never known before. The team creates hope that she may be able to with our help, muster the courage to leave, and start a new life. Courage is the key ingredient to the first step at getting away and leaving the continuous storms of rage that she had to endure. She would no longer have to ride out the storm, but escape it forever. Not everyone survives the storms, but she would.

It was on another Friday that he was drunk again. The beating took place at home, and six days later, waiting for our team to arrive, she gathered up the courage to leave their home and show her face to the team for help. It takes a tremendous amount of strength to make this courageous step forward. It takes getting to the bottom of life sometimes to make that move and to speak to yourself that this is no longer acceptable no matter what happens to me from this point on. Growth starts at that moment and we were praying that God would be with her on this personal journey.

The law in Zambia states that a woman who is abused needs to file a claim against her abuser to a police officer. A written statement is prepared, and the police escort the woman as they did in this case to the hospital for a medical exam and a written report of physical abuse. Upon that document, the police have the ability to apprehend the weasel of a perpetrator and incarcerate him within the time it takes to drive to the jail. There is no trial, no jury, as the broken bones and blackened eyes are the judge. Justice is served within the hour if the police are lucky enough to find and surprise him. It was very swift justice in a country that is relaxed about time and deadlines.

The officers carefully escorted her to our vehicle and drove off across the hills to their destination. The red dust of the village swirled behind the vehicle as other women and men watched the departure. They knew what was going on and I wondered if there was hope for the women who watched. I also wondered if there was fear in the minds of the men who were equally as guilty of the same abuse.

They would soon return with the written medical exam just a few hours later. I could see her face when she returned, still bruised and swollen, but her demeanor had a slight lift and improvement as she was surrounded with the team's support. We cared for her in the pharmacy with vitamins and analgesics. She was being cared for and no longer alone to be controlled by this man. The officers left once again to apprehend her husband in their home just a few kilometers away.

We kept working as she was just one of 497 patients that day all desperately needing care and healing. My next patient had his lower leg wrapped in a dirty rag, weeping with body fluids. A cobra had struck him in the leg and the venom was rapidly eating away at the skin. Wound care station was already backed up, but our nurse there would clean, debride and treat what was a common trauma here in the hills of Baluba. He among others had lost limbs, fingers, and eyesight to the venomous creature that strikes with accurate force and determination to maim or kill.

Before he could get the chance to be treated, my back was to the entrance of the village road that leads to huts, shanties, and desolation. Another soul lost in poverty and alcoholism came staggering in wheeling a worn but heavy hammer, poised in his right hand and ready to strike. "I want to talk to her," he slurred as he came toward me.

Derrick had stepped away for only a moment, and I felt completely vulnerable and in the path of destruction. He was unable to focus on me due to the alcoholic stupor, yet approached with a purpose to get to me without any filter. I moved instinctively and laterally to the edge of the bus, near the second triage station where two other physicians were doing intake histories.

By the time I had moved, the armed guard positioned himself in a location where he could easily move and diffuse the actions of this inebriated man. It was fascinating to watch how they used their expertise in controlling the situation, yet was sensitive to the pitiful condition of this desperate man, wanting to be helped. He broke free of their grasp and staggered near the physician's exam tables, drawing attention from each of them and their patients and interpreters. Derrick was near and without hesitation, apprehended the man who continued to be a threat to our team.

"That's it," I heard Derrick say. "You are going in." Handcuffs were retrieved from his back pocket and with a few clicks the scratched metal bands of confinement were secure on both wrists of the man. The hammer dropped to the ground, no longer a threat. As it would be, and was in the past, we now had another prisoner, destined for jail. The back door of our vehicle opened, and in goes our soon to be jail bird. *Another day at the clinic*, I thought. *It's just another day with much to be thankful for.*

I could see that the officers were pleased in the arrest that they had made. I was pleased to see that justice was so swift. I was honored to be among such strong men who were not intimidated by evil, and were opposed to violence against women. They were trained and willing to do the right thing to bring it to a halt.

It was encouraging to see men who did not approve of abuse, and who honored safety and peace. I was in Africa, on the other side of the world, away from my home, my family, and yet, I felt at home, safe and so validated in life. One woman was saved, one family was free from abuse, and children would never have to witness that violence in that home again.

Baluba is a rough place, and on any day at any time, it is filled with interesting cases, trauma, disease, and extreme poverty. We were about to close the clinic as the sun was setting over the hills of the village, making the area now an even more dangerous place to be. My last patient of the day came quietly over to me complaining of a cough. I looked at her and saw that Hallmark look of eyes lowered to the ground, void of value and lacking all confidence.

"What else is wrong besides your cough?" I asked through my interpreter.

She hesitated, looking side to side as though perhaps she could escape the question. I saw her look around her to see if she was being watched. She slowly lifted the back of her shirt revealing a deep cut that ran from the top of her shoulder blade to her waist. The wound was only a few days old, and obviously was still very painful.

"Who did this to you and what did he use?" I asked in the gentlest tone that I could as not to threaten her state of insecurity any more than it was. I had to repeat the question again, as she was reluctant to answer me.

Her case was no different than the countless other abuse cases we've dealt with: Husband gets paid, gets drunk, and abuses his wife. This time, he almost killed her as the knife he used left a deep wound. If this would have been her front, her neck, or her face, she could have been killed easily.

I took down all the necessary information, date of attack, location, and age of patient and motioned for Derrick and the other armed guard to come over and see the evidence of the domestic abuse. We would file a formal complaint should she agree. I counseled her and warned her that this dangerous aggression against her won't be the last, and the next blow could kill her. She nodded and hung her head lower, agreeing to the warning we had given.

She had been beaten before and had gathered up enough courage to come to the clinic, knowing that we traveled with armed guards, and was willing to get some help. The officers took down a statement and along with Dr. Henry, we wrote our physical and medical findings with the diagnoses: "Knife wound the length of the back observed secondary to domestic abuse."

Our officers, with the direction of Derrick, took off in our vehicle once the report was complete, having the current location of the husband who had inflicted the violent abuse. It was their plan to surprise him quickly, cuff him and let him know of his offense that leads to his arrest. The mission this time was swift and accurate. Our guard, Derrick, and one prisoner came back in a matter of a few minutes. The woman's husband cuffed and now under arrest, was being transported in the back of our vehicle.

The car stopped abruptly near my triage station where I was still tending to the woman and taking her history. From the corner of my eye I saw the guards exit from the vehicle with a pathetic coward of a man about to stand up to be arrested for his abusive terror on his wife.

"What do you want me to do with him, Madam?" asked Derrick as he held the cowering man by the scruff of his shirt.

I knew it was not for me to say, as the law already dictated this abuser's destiny, but I had the pleasure of responding. "Put him in jail and get him away from us."

I looked across the dirt laden clinic at the woman sitting on our bench who had been abused by this man. She sat there with little other than her worn clothes and the small clothe in her hand. She held her head and eyes down, glancing only when she thought she could, still fearful of his violent actions. Her fear was palpable. Her abuser was arrogant, brazen and over confident of his actions.

Derrick ushered the prisoner to the back of our vehicle, secured the back hatch, and they were gone, dust trailing the car, and tail lights dwindling into the darkness. *Another day at the clinic*, I thought. *Another abuser was removed and off the streets. It was just another day here in Zambia.*

Security is of utmost importance not only in the clinics, protecting the teams, but also throughout the days and nights of our absence. Derrick is responsible for it all and keeps us safe, anticipating our arrival, protects us during out stay, and secures our exit from the country.

It was reported to me some time ago that we had some problems again with a staff member. Apparently one employee had a past history of theft involving an armed hitman, carrying out armed robbery on this person's behalf. Injuries from the hit were reported and a large amount of money was missing. Interestingly enough the person involved did not feel the amount was enough and took it to a "magician" in hopes of having the money multiplied. As predicted, the magician and the money did a disappearing act instead of multiplying the funds. The case was not solved and the money was never recovered. The employee is no longer with us.

Above all the criminals, abuse and chaos, there remains an outstanding young man, who sees evil in the world and thwarts its existence. One life at a time, one child at a time, we are all being protected by this astonishing guardian of our safety. The world is ours to care for.

Thank you, Derrick. God is not done with you yet. I am convinced of that.

On Business

It was November of this past year, and I felt the need to return to Africa. The rains had not started yet, but the extreme heat, humidity, and afternoon gusts of threatening winds made each day difficult to keep up the fast pace that we were used to. The evenings only cooled down enough to get some rest.

There were many things that needed to be tended to with the staff, and with the land that was now being threatened to be taken over. Eyes were on our property as the value of the area had risen over the past few years. I had wired money over the week before we arrived and had a fence installed around the entire perimeter of the land. Our staff built two small homes with the brick makers that we bought and used the anthill mounds from our property for homemade bricks. Our guards watched the property around the clock for any trespassers.

Our children in the seventh grade were going to graduate this week. Over 400 people were to attend - including the minister of education and various leaders in the community. Business relationships needed to be secured for advancement of our mission. I had missed Africa and the people and was so glad to be back on African soil.

Staff meetings needed to be done, along with labor law compliance meetings. My time there is never enough and the days are too short, the weeks fly by and more is needed of me. There is pressure to return, like a piece of coal in the process of becoming a diamond. The process is never complete until a beautiful conclusion is completed. I still have work to do and Africa pulls me like a strong magnet. The other pull is for my family here of which remains my greatest love. The commute will continue as the devotion to both remains so powerful. I have struggled with the challenge, and strive for the scales to balance.

Our airline tickets were purchased and Gil, Dr. Henry, and I were to fly over for a week, attend the fifth seventh grade graduation, do home visits, complete the work with the Ndola Rotary, and address staff issues that needed attention. Our agenda was set, I had a sitter for my search dogs at my home and bags full of supplies for our school were packed.

I opened my e-mail in the morning around 6:30 a.m. as I usually do, and found an e-mail from Derrick that was short and profound. *"Dear Madam,*

The Zambian government has confirmed the death of President Michael Sata in London, in a live address by Secretary to Cabinet Dr. Roland Msiska and Vice President Guy Scott has been appointed to act as President of Zambia.

Blessings,

Derrick."

The death of the president was shocking, and marked the third president to die in office since the beginning of our mission for the poor in Zambia fourteen years ago.

Derrick called shortly after reading his e-mail and expressed his great concern for our travel to the country due to the potential of political unrest.

"I cannot guarantee your safety, Madam while you are here. If I can't do that, I am not doing my job," he explained.

"Well, I am not afraid to come in." I quickly responded to his concerns.

"That is what we thought and were afraid of," he said.

I had to smile, as I felt that I continue to be his challenge, not intentionally, but it was just the way that it was.

"I have to insist Madam that you not come to the country. All of the police in the country have been ordered to be on standby for deployment in the event of unrest. I am also on stand by and cannot be with you if I was deployed by the police," he continued.

Out of respect for Derrick and all he's done for me and OMNI, I had to listen to his recommendations and comply. As much as I wanted to defy that decision, I agreed that we would cancel our business trip to Zambia.

Dr. Henry and Gil who were going to travel with me agreed that it would be in our best interest to not travel at this time, despite the graduation taking place next week, and our travel plans secured. Everyone cancelled their plans to travel, but I kept our international flights scheduled, just in case.

Three days later, Derrick called again, to say that the tensions on the ground had lessened, but were not completely resolved.

"I still want to come in, and with your help, we can do this," I declared. "Please go to the chief of police and ask if he can release you from being on the list for deployment while I am there."

I waited for another day, talking to Dr. Henry several times and going over our options if this would not work. We both felt that we needed to make this trip. Without it, time would lapse and the staff issues and efforts for progress would deteriorate.

The message came back the following day that Derrick would be off the deployment list for a national crisis, and we were free to come in. The national police would assign an armed guard as well to us for the week. Derrick felt assured that our assignment of a police officer would be one of quality.

We had only a few days to prepare for our departure, so changing schedules and connecting flights became a slight challenge, but doable. Gil had, unfortunately, changed plans here that did not allow her to travel out of the country, so Henry and I had to make the decision to go ahead, or cancel the business trip all together. There was so much work that needed to be done in Zambia, and our children would be graduating in just a few days. We decided to make the trip, leaving DC on the evening flight that would get us to our destination in thirty-six hours.

Over the years, I have become so very grateful for Dr. Henry. He has been a mentor, a leader, and a very dear friend. His strength of character is solid and I am a better person for having known him and worked with him in various challenging settings. The years have done well by him and I look to him more and more for this work that we have been called to do. He is a faithful servant and God must be so very pleased with him.

We flew in arriving through South Africa on a Monday. Teddy met us at the small airport, and because we had no medications to declare, we were free to come through customs rather quickly. Outside of the tin airport, was our assigned guard in uniform and complete with his AK47 rifle. He was known to us, and I felt comfortable once again. It felt like we were home.

The following day, the country declared a day of official mourning as the presidential funeral was taking place in the capital hours to our south. Almost all countries in the continent of Africa sent their president and his entourage to the funeral. Airspace was closed over the large stadium that housed the funeral service and leaders from various countries paid their respect in forms of speeches, traditional music and dedications to a well-loved President of the people of Zambia. Letters, prayers, and tributes to Zambia's beloved president were presented all day as the people who had means could watch on televisions.

It was a solemn day all around. The staff at the small hotel that we stayed in lingered around the television that stayed on through the day in the lobby. Reverence was paid as the national anthem played, singers from around the country sang in homage to their fallen president. Flags in the country flew at half-mast as businesses, schools, and all activities closed in respect for this revered President now being laid to rest in the cemetery in the capital of the country. We felt their sense of loss as well.

The following morning, businesses opened and the country felt the need to carry on without their beloved man, leader for the poor and champion for those who had no voice. We had to prepare for the graduation of the fifth successful class having accomplished all requirements and passing their exams.

I asked to travel to Baluba the Congolese Refugee village that had at one point been our challenge, yet because of the dear people there, has become one of my favorite places. Violence is present. Disease and disorder is there, but there are people who appreciate the love and care that OMNI has given.

I wanted to see little Karen, the child that OMNI saved eight years ago from starvation. Her grandmother was her guardian and her angel her on earth. Karen's mother left when she was critically ill despite our efforts to help them bond. We used every teaching skill we had to connect the mother to her child, but it was not in her make up. She now lives somewhere nearby but is not involved in her child's life.

We drove down the dirt road through the familiar mud shacks, thugs drinking local brew, and children afraid of a white face. We passed the skinny chickens, goats, babies being bathed in dirty water for the world to see, and endless poverty. We approached the building that OMNI conducts our annual medical clinic and passed further up the road to a dirt path. This was the landmark that we would stop the vehicle and walk to the huts in front of us.

It was so hot that day, maybe in the lower 90s and every step seemed an effort. Dr. Henry and I were still feeling the effects of jet lag and perhaps lack of water. We had to move forward and see if Karen was there.

Under a tree a little woman slept on the dirt in the shade. She had no ground mat or pillow to cradle her head. It was the faithful grandmother of Karen. She quickly got up and straightened her shetange that wrapped her small short frame, and tried to present herself to her guests. She came to me and hugged me, and shook Dr. Henry's hand as she remembered quickly who we were.

Derrick asked on our behalf about little Karen and we were told that she was down at the river swimming with the children to keep cool. The day was so very hot and humid and the air was heavy with odors that were not pleasant. We walked back to the car through the dirt yards of neighbors and stepped over what seemed to be pieces of garbage of unknown origin. We drove a short distance then walked down to the green reeds and flowing water that created the source of comfort for the children during this muggy rainy, hot season.

Karen came running as fast as she could from the river on the dirt path, barefoot and full of energy and jumped into my arms. The children that she was with followed in her path and were hesitant until they saw her obvious familiarity with us. It was a great moment again in our trip and in my life. Dr. Henry and I were surrounded by the very reason that we were there: impoverished children in need.

Typically, as children gather and feel safe, more and more come and want to be in on the action. Small ones would wiggle their way to our sides and larger ones would push them away to be in the core of the crowd. Smiles were everywhere. How simple and how precious they were.

We took her back to her grandmother who was waiting at the withering hut down the road from the river. The children loaded into the back of our pickup and all sat down on the floor of the truck bed as we slowly sent down the dirt road. Walking with children attached to both hands we made it to the shack that was home to Karen, her grandmother and six other children. The handmade bricks had cracked leaving large gaps in the corner structure of the house. The roof sagged and was rotting from many rainy seasons. The space was inadequate for the family, and inadequate for the next rainy season.

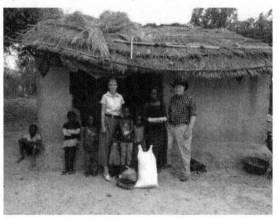

Karen's grandmother's house.

It was clear that a new roof was needed and Dr. Henry and I agreed to split the cost as we looked at the rotten grass roof. Derrick walked around the structure and came back with the conclusion that it was not safe enough to hold a new roof. A new house was needed, or the entire building could collapse on the family during the first heavy rain.

"Go ahead and start the brick making," I confirmed. I would find donors and we will build Karen a new home. Karen had been with OMNI for many years, and we had saved her life. It was time to do more.

The message was delivered to the grandmother who immediately put her worn brown hands together, clapping in appreciation. We got a group hug from the children and the grandmother before we left. We walked away from the hut, through the few chickens that were running free and past the sea of other needs within our reach. It was one family, one child, and we were going to make a difference and provide for them a modest home that would be a safe haven.

A text was sent from me to the states to Jon to ask for a plea of support to be posted on our web site. We would build a home for Karen and her family. Building here would begin on Monday. The building project was based on faith that it would be supported by generous donors.

The following morning, we had more work to do, and the day would be filled from sun up to sun down. We met with the owner of the largest pharmacy in town and discussed our needs for the following medical mission. Banking was done in the alley next to the shops downtown. Fabric was purchased in the shop owned by a family from India. We had purchased fabrics there for many years, and the procedure was always the same. I marveled at the cash flow and the hand written receipts. Business was important there and by our observation was doing well.

Back at the OMNI School, the women of the school and village had been preparing chickens, potatoes, and vegetables to serve the families of the graduates and those of the community that would attend this grand ceremony.

Dr. Henry and I were at the disposal of our guard and headmaster as the preparations had to be tended to. We only have one vehicle, so the choices were to be left behind or go with the crew and gather the supplies for the celebration. We purchased forty bags of potatoes, forty chickens, and found ourselves at various beverage companies while we watched cases of Fanta, the local orange drink, and Coca-Cola being loaded by hand with a dolly motorized by thin nationals pushing the cumbersome loads to the back of our truck. The heat was stifling and we were dehydrated despite the volumes of delicious and coveted liquids in our possession.

One of our stops was at the national police guard stations so that we could rent tents to shield the crowds from the hot sun. Our vehicle was allowed entrance into the secured gates of the compound. Once inside, a uniformed guard immediately came to the driver's side of the vehicle and asked for our reason for arrival to the compound. Our logo on the car, OMNI signaled that we were at least registered in the country and had some legitimization.

The armed officer leaned into the vehicle and asked for the driver's license and country equivalent of a passport of our headmaster Teddy.

"We are coming to rent the tents for our gradation for OMNI. We have rented from you for the past five years," Teddy said.

"Have the white people in the back exit and go out of this compound," said the officer.

Our car backed out of the secured gates, and we were ushered out of the vehicle to stand under a tree on the exterior of the compound. I felt the blunt accost of discrimination that I have not experienced previously and realized at that moment what it was like to be separated and demeaned as a minority. This is what I stood up for years ago for the African Americans in my own country. I always felt we were equal and felt the sting and heavy burden that racism carries. Now we were the ones who were not allowed to enter, not allowed to be part of a very simple task because of the color of our skin in an African country. How ironic and poignant. It is wrong, and the antidote along with love of man will need to include education and acceptance. We are people of this world, not different, not more or less because of the shade of our skin, or eye color or continent of origin. We are all people who inhabit this globe of ours. Each and every life is precious.

A tall wall was the only thing that separated us from the hot sun and the entrance of the compound. We moved to a tree nearby for shade and the armed guard circled around us. Within minutes, another guard donning a different uniform and of higher rank came out to inspect the detainees. My business card was presented to each officer, as well as Dr. Henry's card. I resorted to my pristine Zambian respect and manners to greet those in authority.

Time passed, guards remained, and eventually there came a few apologies for protocol for denial of entrance into a military compound. I understood more that they were aware of. I was in their country and was compliant of the rules being enforced. I had to be.

Once our truck backed out of the armed gate that surrounded the military compound, Teddy backed up and parked within a few yards of the entrance to the base. Dr. Henry and I walked to the truck to get into the back row and leave.

A man in street clothes approached me and asked if I remember him. I could not place him from his casual street attire, but had flashbacks of his face. He was a tall, strong looking man in his mid-thirties and well groomed. He spoke with a deep voice that was equally strong. "I was your guard when you arrested the man years ago for auto theft," He said.

I knew the unusual situation he referred to and had vivid images of him as he drove the white run down car that went through the town on a sting to arrest Felton. How history has a way of circling around and keeping us connected. What a small world. He threw his jacket over his shoulder and walked away looking back just a few feet from me. "I hope that we will work together again someday," he said with a smile.

"Indeed, we may just do that," I replied.

We left untouched and unscathed and drove through the town to prepare for the graduation of the children at the OMNI School.

"There may be the next future president of this country waiting for us. The future of this country is in their hands," I said to Henry.

The gigantic crimson Africa sun was just starting its progressive descent over the smoke that was rising from the tiny village huts. Our truck turned down the well-traveled gravel road that no so long ago was only a rugged dirt trail to the OMNI village.

I received this e-mail today from Zambia:

Hi Karen,

Greetings to you and the family and the OMNI Team. Karen it's with deep regret to inform you that Mildred the lady you so much supported when you came to Zambia and in particular Maurigrace Schools passed on to be with the Lord on the 7th of March 2015, she was buried in Lusaka on the 10th of March 2015. I attended the burial. If you recall this is the lady you visited. She served Maurigrace faithfully until the time she left to join pastoral work in Grace Ministries Church in Zambia to which still you were a great support until she graduated from Seminary. Maurice and myself we shall live to remember her good works as we do for you. God bless you so much.

Yours for Christ sake,
Everlyne-
Maurigrace Schools

The passing of Mildred felt like the passing of a miracle. Faith and four dollars had given a widow and her children a new and better life. The small amount of money given by some elderly woman years ago had far surpassed our expectations and hope. It is not the amount, similar to the widow's mite in Luke 21. It was her faith and willingness to give all that she had that created the miracle for Mildred.

The following day, I received more news about Mildred.

Karen,

Thanks for your response Karen. She died from low blood levels, in December last year during her bout of malaria. I personally suspected the treatment was not comprehensive and she quickly reported for duty. She was chosen to pastor a church in eastern province of Zambia about eight hours drive from Lusaka and eleven hours from Ndola. I never had chance to visit her since four years when her church transferred her from Lusaka immediately she remarried. I had kept contact with her by means of mobile phone.

Shalom
Yours for Christ sake,
Everlyn

Mildred,

Rest in peace and know that you served well. Your work was
acknowledged and recognized by many. The woman who thought she
could not make an impact by donating $4.00 to Africa would be so proud
of you. We thank God for your service and for your faith to serve in His
name. Rest well faithful woman, good mother and friend. You were brave
and faithful. Your service was not in vain.

Love,
Karen

The following week, another dreaded and unexpected e-mail
came in from Teddy.

Karen,
I regret to inform you, mum, that Grace has died and her burial will be
tomorrow.
Regards,
Teddy

The e-mail was so short and left no details.

Teddy had to deliver such painful news about Grace. He had
successfully led the OMNI School the entire time that Grace had
attended. He had been the firsthand witness of impoverished children,
broken, starving and without hope, passing through our gates and

leaving with an education, healthy bodies, and strengthened spirits. He had been honored by OMNI as teacher of the year, and had grown as a man of true leadership. His maturity and compassion was being refined once again by the death of Grace.

Grace graduated in the first class almost five years ago, and did not have the chance to get her hip surgically corrected. She had become pregnant, and, during the difficult delivery, had been unable to deliver her baby vaginally. She was taken to the operating arena at the general hospital in town. Both she and her baby died during that surgery, and were buried together the following day. Once again, our hearts were broken at the loss of this young woman and her precious baby. The news was devastating.

The past in Zambia always seems to come forward to the present day, and people that I thought would be gone from our lives reappear unexpectedly from time to time.

Cutter e-mailed me a couple of days ago, and after wishing me well asked that I would sponsor his daughter in college as things were financially tight there. He had suffered a stroke a couple of years after his scam project where he stole sand from the OMNI site. After being bedridden as a young man, and unable to work, his wife was carrying the financial burden of the family's needs. She apparently was doing a good job as the children had made their way through high school and now were enrolled in a local college.

"Congratulations Felton on the success of your daughter. I am sure that you are very proud of her. Due to recent financial changes here, I am unable to assist you. Please greet your wife for me," I replied.

It's really too bad that he didn't save all the money that he took from us as it would have come in handy for his family right now. Well, I am sure that I will hear from him again when he needs something.

This week was also interesting in hearing about people's past. This time an e-mail came from Derrick with the following information:

Dear Madam,

I received reliable information about our accountant does not have a clean record background were accounting is concerned, Two years ago an accountant was killed at a place of employment after two gunmen opened fire onto the Hilux that was carrying money from the bank in town to the work HQ in Ndola that was meant to pay salaries for employees but Police from Twapia police station managed to shot the gun men in the legs and took them into custody were the gun men reviewed that He was part of the people who planned for the attack together with other accountants after they misappropriated funds at his work place and wanted to recover the money. He was covered and was not arrested and the matter died a natural death.

After a few months the accountant and the friends decided to find means of which they could recover the money before top management could request for a financial report. This time a huge sum of money amounting to K 300, 000 went missing at his work place of which the accountant and his friends took the money to a magician in order for him to double the money using magic and be able to recover the misappropriated funds but the magician disappeared after receiving the said monies.

Three accountants were arrested by police to help with investigations and our former accountant was suspended from work to allow police investigate the matter without interference. Even this time around he was mentioned by his work mates that he was part of the deal but his mother having a top position at sited place of employment managed to cover the accountant and he was returned back at work. The accountant is dangerous. The firearm that was used in the attack was said to be from the Congo.

I wait for your directions.

In His Service,
Derrick

My response was clear and swift.

Termination is in order. I trust that you will handle this well and appropriately.

I wondered where the magician was now...

Our Land

My cell phone rang at 4:20 a.m. the following morning. I knew it must be a serious situation that needed my attention.

"OMNI has been summoned to the city council and questioned and accused of encroaching on land that was not ours," he reported. "We need the land title, the map demarcation and a letter of intent by fifteen hours. They also want to see the president of OMNI now."

It was early and still dark here, but I started scanning documents, and sending to Derrick to present to the council. It was interesting that now, after nine years of occupying the land, developing a large school with 210 students, over twenty staff, bore holes, laying hens and crops that the council was eyeing our land. We had spent thousands of dollars just this year putting up a fence around the entire seventeen hectors and building larger corner beacons to establish property demarcation.

The road to our property was a lonely unleveled dirt path nine years ago, and was now a well-traveled gravel road to reach the village of George. What made this long stretch now desirable was the multimillion dollar soccer stadium that was built just a few miles away in memory of past president Mwanasawa. Homes, businesses, and lodges had popped up all around in anticipation of increased traffic and income. Our children's village now sits on very valuable land for those who have an eye for a prosperous business endeavor.

Fifteen years ago, OMNI was created with nothing but a vision and prayers that God would be with us through it all. Today sixty acres of African soil is home to the OMNI school in George. I have made forty-two trips to Africa and wait to go back soon. Our school educates 206 children who without our care could not afford to be educated due to their extreme poverty. We have eight fantastic teachers who have been educated to higher standards thanks to OMNI. There stands a beautiful building named after Morgan Harrington that has three classrooms and embraces the educational efforts of three grades. The cafeteria holds four more classrooms, but we are bursting at the seams in need of more space.

Wonderful men and women fill the teacher's offices, ready to work daily to educate our children. The office of the accountant is filled once again.

Across the campus was the agricultural area where lush green crops grow to supplement the food program. The hen house has been expanded and now holds 200 laying hens, giving eggs daily to boost and augment the protein needs of the children. A new cafeteria building donated by a private donor through the help of the Ndola Rotary is the site where the nutritious meals are prepared each day for the students. Our guard station is manned around the clock with security hired from local men needing work.

On the two corners closest to the George compound stood two small homes now occupied by one of our guards and the other by Jane and her children. A grinding mill is located on the other side of the campus allowing villagers to grind the corn from their harvests.

Three bore holes with towers and tanks provide clean potable water for our children, staff and for villagers thanks to grants from churches here in the U.S. The administration building holds offices for the staff, computers, lesson planners, and up-to-date textbooks filled the shelves, thanks to generous donors.

Most importantly, happy children wearing red shirts embossed with the OMNI logo and blue pants or skirts that Teddy sewed, filled the campus. Everyone has shoes, mosquito nets at home to prevent malaria, and access to health care. Beautiful voices and music can be heard down the road when our kids sing songs. Smiles are everywhere, and there is hope. This is where we have come, and there is more to do.

Thirty-seven duffels filled with medications and supplies for Africa are packed, labeled, inventoried, and waiting like ducks in a row to be loaded onto the trailer and taken to Africa with the medical team once again. Donor's hearts have been touched in various ways that prompted them to give a monetary donation, medications that were needed, crutches, canes, new blankets, and hats. St. John Lutheran church made 600 care kits for the children at the school providing them with bare necessities like soap, washcloths, toothbrushes, and paste.

A woman in town made over 200 birthing kits that will save the life of a mother and her baby and only costs $1.60 each. Each kit contains a piece of plastic for the mother to lay on during the delivery, a bar of soap, a pair of plastic gloves, string for the cord, a razor blade to cut the cord, and a candle and matches in the event of a night birth. A small washcloth is included to wipe off the baby, a simple thing yet no one has these in their home. This year, we will be adding erythromycin eye ointment that will prevent blindness in newborn babies. With the additional kits we had in stock, over 1,000 pregnant women and their babies will be helped on this mission.

Ladies from the bible study donated over 100 tubes of antibiotic ointment for the pharmacy. Tropical wounds that would have developed into limb threatening conditions will be cured. One small gesture can save a life and does. I remain grateful.

We received a $25,000 donor challenge from one of our supporters to build another wing identical to the Morgan Harrington Wing. Money is coming in slowly. We desperately need more classrooms and we need to keep showing progress on the land.

This all went through my mind as I listened to the details of the threat to our land.

I have no problem or hesitation supplying our official documents on demand for review, however, my presence at this meeting was not possible or reasonable. Derrick did a fine job presenting our title papers and all documents that were demanded of us in a short period of time. He also was comfortable standing up asking serious questions of those who had a personal interest in snatching our land.

"My president will not be in the country until July, and you can make an appointment with her at that time," he concluded.

The discussion and interrogation for the moment was over, and our land was safe for now.

Epilogue

It was just past July, and, again, I found my way down the dirt path through the resting corn fields, waiting for new seeds to be planted. The fields were dormant, having produced all that they could in their season.

Smoke slowly escaped from the weathered wooden cooking structure next to Felishi's hut. Chickens walked past me, and the house seemed quiet. Two young women exited from her home, staring at me and back again.

I wanted to see her and give her the picture of us laughing together that last time we saw each other.

Felishi's daughter slowly began, "Felishi was asking for you to come and get her. In her final hours, she was asking for you. She died in October just two months after you left."

My heart felt heavy... sad... that she had died. Yet, I gave thanks that she lived well beyond the years that Africa normally allows.

"I'll come and find you, Felishi and take you with me, when my work is done," I said aloud. I could smell the smoke and the African earth as I walked down the narrow path back to our vehicle.

There will be more work in July, and I am not yet done.

CPSIA information can be obtained
at www.ICGtesting.com
Printed in the USA
FSOW04n1715051116
27015FS